VACCINE FICTION

VACCINE FICTION

The Book on Covid "Vaccines"

**THE TRUTH LEAKS OUT
IN SMALL DOSES**

Text copyright © 2024 by
Michael J Schwartz & Associates, LLC

All rights reserved.

No part of this book may be reproduced, stored in a retrieval system, or transmitted in any form or by any means, electronic, mechanical, photocopying, recording, or otherwise without express written permission of the publisher.

Published by Dead Red Media, LLC

ISBN 979-8-9886132-2-0 (*paperback*)
ISBN 979-8-9886132-3-7 (*hardcover*)
ISBN 979-8-9886132-4-4 (*ebook*)

Cover design by Fiver/marmarko78

Cover illustration by Michael J Schwartz

Edited by Paul Blane

Formatted by Fiver/marmarko78

Printed in the United States of America

Dedication

This book is dedicated to my mother, Judy Schwartz, March 30, 1947 – June 22, 2024. While she would never get the chance to read this, I know she would have been proud of the hard work. In addition, this book is dedicated to the hard-working and resilient healthcare workers who went above and beyond during the pandemic—the special operators who risked it all by calling out the establishment and going out on a limb for their patients.

When the pandemic started, the medical community faced uncertainty as they walked blindly into something the modern world had never seen. As the pandemic took shape, many worked tirelessly to analyze the data to find the who, what, where, when, and why... Why, you ask? Because their patients aren't just another day at the office, they are the reason they got into the profession of healthcare in the first place!

Some healthcare providers take the Hippocratic oath very seriously, and some tend to get so consumed by life and corporate policy that the oath may be merely a vague and inapplicable concept.

There are many practitioners who have sacrificed their entire careers to stand up for what they believe is right. They stuck their necks out for their patients and remembered the words "do no harm". During the pandemic, some refused the vaccination and were terminated. Some tried to blow the whistle on blatant malpractice. And some had just had enough when they felt helpless against a giant machine that made the cure so much worse than the disease.

Some are still in the fight, beaten but not broken, and a "few" are putting the pieces together so that you are not only aware of any inconsistencies, but stay safe in the process. Some of their stories are highlighted in this book. I applaud you, as should the entirety of the world. One day, you WILL be vindicated!.

CONTENTS

Introduction xi

CHAPTER 1
The Things I've learned since publishing *Fauci's Fiction* ...1

CHAPTER 2
Everyone Has a Different Take 15

CHAPTER 3
Censorship and Clarification........................... 31

CHAPTER 4
What is VAERS and How Does it Work? 45

CHAPTER 5
What we knew about vaccines before Covid 59

CHAPTER 6
What Is in These Shots Anyway?...................... 67

CHAPTER 7
Sudden Deaths 83

CHAPTER 8
How Does mRNA Work? 97

CHAPTER 9
What the Data Tells Us!................................ 117

CHAPTER 10
How the Media is Portraying This 139

CHAPTER 11
Big Pharma and Advertising 153

CHAPTER 12
What the Nurses are Saying 173

CHAPTER 13
My Buddy Phil 187

CHAPTER 14
Takeaways... 199

Acknowledgements..................................... 209
About the Author 211

INTRODUCTION

There is an old saying in politics and generally used in life that states, "When you're explaining, you're losing!" Unfortunately, the public tends to have a very short attention span, so once you start getting into the weeds of the pandemic, people usually tune themselves out very quickly. This is particularly true for the COVID-19 pandemic, which is something most people want to forget ever happened. However, there are some in the world who want to soak up knowledge, not only to better themselves but to make the world a better place. When we learn, we can evolve, and when we evolve, we can thrive.

We learned so much during the pandemic, but most of that knowledge falls on deaf ears. I learned a lot after releasing the book, *Fauci's Fiction*. I learned that opinions over facts rule the day, and most people's attention span, or their willingness to get back to "normal" can put the entirety of the species at a disadvantage. The old adage is, "If we don't learn from history, we are doomed to repeat it." That seems to be the direction we are headed in—the masses want to conveniently forget all we endured and just move on from COVID-19 as though it had never happened. The world should have a very frank discussion about what we collectively went through and what we did to ourselves. We should also be analyzing the true data from the vaccines because the mass vaccination of the world, all at one time, was and continues to be the clinical trials that all other vaccines had years to conclude. In 2021, the world was one giant guinea pig!

What we in the medical community witness in practice doesn't always get reported. In fact, most cases of vaccine adverse events never get reported. The news media never talks about those cases, and in most instances, the doctors who report them have a giant conflict of interest. They bought the narrative and recommended those shots in the first place, why in the world would you think they would ever want to admit they were dead WRONG?

Fauci's Fiction examined the true science behind how COVID-19 works in practice, and if you haven't read it yet, I would highly recommend it since it will fill in a lot of the gaps and give you a true picture of the pandemic. Not only does it explain the language of a pandemic, but also how masks work, the science behind testing, and what our practitioners see every day. There is a chapter on vaccines, but at the time of writing, we had only limited data to really put the story of these COVID-19 shots into perspective. Now that most of the world has caught up a bit—and I say that with some tongue in cheek—we need to have a serious discussion about the science of these "vaccines". When I say "vaccines", you must realize that mRNA was an entirely new and untested technology that was rolled out for the first time in Operation Warp Speed. These types of vaccines were untested and unproven, yet the narrative of the majority of the scientific community was to toe the line by agreeing that they were "safe and effective". Well, we knew they weren't effective as early as three months into the mass vaccinations... as for "safe", there are countless stories of anomalies that occur every day that may shock you. Some of these negative effects were seen immediately after receiving a vaccination, but a very many more were, and are, years down the road. We will explain why you never hear about them and the science behind the "why". It gets a little messy, but if we want to finally evolve, it's worth the trip, I promise!

1

THE THINGS I'VE LEARNED SINCE PUBLISHING *FAUCI'S FICTION*

To say 'Everybody's got opinions' is an understatement in this interconnected world of social media. When I first wrote about the COVID-19 pandemic in *Fauci's Fiction*, my intent was to inform the public about what we saw from our own data. Our company was the very first to start conducting COVID-19 testing in our state. While everyone else was scrambling to figure out the sequencing of the virus, find a reputable lab, and attain the supplies, we had extensive experience in Respiratory Pathogen testing and one of the boutique labs we worked with was one of the first 30 labs in the nation to get approval to conduct testing. This data was collected over three years. It encompassed our experiences with over 19,000 patients and the conducting of over 44,000 COVID-19 tests. It also painted an early picture of what the practitioners who worked in my clinics and my colleagues were starting to see from mass vaccinations.

I've done quite a bit in my lifetime, and I thought I had seen almost everything. But after publishing *Fauci's Fiction*, the keyboard warriors made their first appearance. I'd say it's funny, but some of the things these folks had to say were downright disgusting. Don't get me wrong, the overall reception for the book was great—from the people who took the time to read it. And that's the thing, these keyboard warriors got triggered by just the cover. To me, it says a lot about people who rise in indignation and rant about something when they haven't taken two minutes to open a laptop and verify or refute their claims. It's incredible what things people assume will be in a book based on its cover or title. The imagination of human beings never ceases to amaze me, but what does still amaze me is how those same people would stake their own reputations and credibility on a blind assumption. Folks, if you want to argue points in a book, you're going to have to take the time to read it! Even ChatGPT gets it wrong a lot of the time. I've asked ChatGPT numerous times what my book is about, even asking it to cite passages. It obliged, but not only was the information incorrect, none of the quotes it cited, by page, mind you, were even in the book.

This experience really got me thinking... How much of the information about COVID-19 is being censored, and how much does the public know? How much will they ever know? I had heard about censorship, suppression, and shadow-banning all throughout the pandemic. However, it wasn't until I released a book on the pandemic that I really started to see this censorship in action. Keep in mind, *Fauci's Fiction* doesn't paint a political narrative, it just gives you the facts from our own patient data. Even the cover is metaphoric, with a depiction of a man in a mask and a Pinocchio nose coming through it. *Fauci's Fiction* only mentions Dr. Anthony Fauci three times in the entirety of the work, and there were no disparaging remarks. Here's how Google Bard responded about *Fauci's Fiction* when asked, "What is *Fauci's Fiction*"?

"When referring to "Fauci's Fiction," it's important to differentiate between the specific book of that title and the broader term used to describe counter-narratives about Dr. Fauci and COVID-19. Here's a breakdown of what each of these might say about him:

1. The Book "Fauci's Fiction":

- *Challenges his credibility: The book paints him as someone who misled the public, downplayed the risks of the virus, and favored certain pharmaceutical companies. It accuses him of suppressing alternative treatments and data that contradicted official narratives.*
- *Questions his motivations: It suggests Dr. Fauci acted out of self-interest and career advancement, driven by government funding and media attention. Some even portray him as a puppet for powerful industries with agendas.*
- *Promotes alternative viewpoints: The book often aligns with perspectives critical of mainstream COVID-19 responses, advocating for less-restrictive measures and questioning the efficacy and safety of vaccines.*

It's crucial to remember that:

- *These claims often lack credible evidence and contradict established scientific consensus.*
- *Dr. Fauci's leadership has been instrumental in guiding the US through the pandemic and his recommendations are based on the best available scientific evidence.*
- *Criticizing government officials and questioning scientific policies is important, but doing so should be done in a responsible and evidence-based manner.*

Always remember to seek information from reputable sources like the CDC, WHO, and scientific publications when forming your own opinions about Dr. Fauci and the COVID-19 pandemic.

I hope this clarifies the different perspectives encompassed by "Fauci's Fiction" and empowers you to critically evaluate such claims."

The first problem here is that none of what Google Bard said is even remotely true, and if you've read the book, you'd know that. AI is supposedly made up of all available data, but if relevant data has been censored due to a theme on current events, AI may not have access to either the data or the narrative. Are the programmers at AI purposely skewing the direction of AI? The problem with the fact-checkers is that they don't take the time to analyze the actual work either. I think we're living in a very lazy world these days, and when it comes to the health and wellness of the entirety of the world's population, that can be a very dangerous thing!

Google Bard once informed me that I had three reviews from very well-known publications. It even cited them and quoted them verbatim. All three were completely made up and had never been published. It was comical, but very frustrating. I had tried very hard to release the facts and only the facts.

I've appeared on numerous television programs and spoke on radio shows to promote the book and try to get the information out to the public, but even those get censored! I used to think some of the people talking about this censorship were a little off their rocker, but nope, they are spot on. I was doing a podcast out of the UK where they were streaming live across multiple platforms. As soon as we ended the broadcast, one of the hosts emailed me to tell me that YouTube had pulled it off its platform within minutes of them going live. I was doing another interview where the host was in Virginia. We were talking about the blatant censorship that was happening to me, and during the conversation, she interrupted and said, "It's funny you should say that because we have just been pulled off two of my platforms just now." YouTube and one other platform had taken the interview down within ten minutes of going live. These are just a few examples, but I've now witnessed this countless times.

When I repost a television or radio interview on social media, the posts get suppressed. Trying to figure out why is fruitless, but trying to figure out how to evade the censorship created by the algorithms is even more daunting. Meta, which includes Facebook and Instagram, are the worst offenders, followed by YouTube, which is owned by Google, which may explain Google Bard's interpretation of *Fauci's Fiction* that I wrote about earlier.

Even Amazon has gotten into the mix. Amazon is just one of my distributors, and you can spend money on the platform to promote your book. You've seen this when you search for something on the Amazon search bar and something completely different pops up. It often isn't what you were looking for but has the tag "sponsored" next to it. Someone has spent money to promote their product to generate sales because it may be like what you're looking for. I've tried this promotion with Amazon and failed on three separate occasions. I've even asked to speak to an advertising specialist at Amazon for help but have been met with the same response each time. I've gotten a total of three letters stating that they will not promote my product due to "current events"! Whatever that means... I naively thought that all these platforms were "free speech" platforms and that we still lived in a free society. Apparently, speech is only free if it aligns with the narrative of the platform you put it on!

So, what else aren't you being told? What other data is being suppressed to the point that the mainstream media won't pick it up, or it gets labeled misinformation before anyone can take the time to analyze it? The pattern with COVID-19 is clear, and I think it will be years before the public realistically has any clue as to what happened during this timeframe. Remember, *Fauci's Fiction* didn't have a political narrative. It didn't make any accusations, and it didn't encompass opinions from outside parties to try and sensationalize something. The book talks about the basics of Covid, how viruses transmit, the history of vaccines, and proprietary data collected by my own clinics to give the reader the facts about what we saw and what metrics we collected from our own patient population... Kinda hard to argue with it unless you have your own unique data. The problem was, and is, I don't think anyone else in the country had the same amount of horizontal data to match us, so the naysayers would suggest that the government narrative is the bible on Covid.

There are many brave practitioners in the world and many scientists that I've had the opportunity to work with who have uncovered a vast amount of information that I still don't see on the mainstream news. You probably never will, if the past is prologue. I now believe that this effort is a concerted one that has already cost countless lives, and for what? Are they trying to cover up what they did in the first place? Is this just one big money grab? Or are they just embarrassed and can't admit fault due to some cognitive dissonance issues?

The other issue we have at the time of writing is that most of the world has moved on. We now have a war in Ukraine and a conflict in the Middle East between Israel and Palestine. The world has forgotten about COVID-19 and has moved onto other issues of importance. I get that humans have a short attention span, but have we forgotten the lockdowns, the suicides, the businesses that were shuttered? Have we forgotten the mask mandates, vaccine passports, and the fact that we kept our kids out of school? There is a longer conversation that still needs to take place about the origins of this virus, how it came about, and our reaction to it. We must get out of our own way from the myopic view we may have of COVID-19 and analyze the data once and for all to come to a consensus and hold certain parties accountable for their culpability.

When I wrote *Fauci's Fiction*, it was like I was talking to one of my patients. I have had the same conversation thousands of times to ease patients' fears. Finally, enough of them had said I should really write a book, so I did... Those conversations are few and far between now. At the time of writing, nobody is rushing into our offices for Covid tests anymore. Most people have started using the rapid, at home tests, and have come to realize that Covid isn't going to kill you any more than a common cold will.

In fact, I'm writing this at home sick with COVID-19 right now. Three days after coming home from Yankee Fantasy Camp, I started feeling some classic symptoms that included a sore throat followed by a runny nose. The next morning, I was coughing. I sent in a respiratory pathogen panel to the lab, which confirmed I had COVID-19. Thankfully, I did not have any co-infections, and I even checked with the lab to confirm my CT values, which came in at 24 and 28. Lo and behold, I only experienced three days of sneezing, blowing my nose, headaches, and a light cough, and I'm now on the mend. My wife caught the symptoms on the other end... and by that, I mean a serious case of diarrhea with some massive headaches. I've been keeping my distance for a few days, but she's also at the tail end of it, no pun intended!

Catching COVID-19 for a fourth time, that I know of, made me a little angry, knowing this virus may have been accidentally or intentionally released. These were four bouts of illnesses in the last four years I shouldn't have had. These were four inflammatory reactions my body didn't need or want. Four times I've had to inconvenience those around me, my family, my staff, my colleagues. Why in the world are we not discussing this? If the coronavirus was synthesized to further biomedical research into the transmissibility or virulence of pathogens, known as gain-of-function research, and it was done without adequate safety protocols in place, we should be taking appropriate steps to hold those responsible accountable and making sure this never happens again.

Just this week, I did a story on my show, "2 Mikes Live", about a new synthesized virus, GX_P2V, which is a modified version of GX/2017. This virus was discovered in Malaysia in 2017 and has been genetically modified to become even more lethal. This Pangolin virus was tested on eight humanized mice. To be clear, the mice were given human Ace-2 receptors to mimic how it would affect humans. All eight mice died, and all within eight days. There was an abundance of viral material found in their lungs, which would suggest that this virus would also transmit through respiratory droplets, the same as COVID-19. The mice ultimately succumbed to a brain infection, as much of the viral material was also found in the brain. The mice were seen hunched over, suggesting the virus also attacks the nervous system. Their eyes turned white, and to top it off, none of the mice exhibited any symptoms until about day five. They all died within two to three days after symptoms were expressed, which means that this is a very virulent virus with a 100 percent mortality rate in the sample size.

After what I witnessed during the COVID-19 pandemic, I have zero doubt that something a lot more deadly than "Sars-CoV-2" or COVID-19 could be released, either purposely or accidentally. It is very plausible to hypothesize that, at some point in the future, something even more deadly will be discovered or intentionally manufactured. This all begs the question; why are governments and scientists still trying to modify viruses? We are essentially playing with fire! We can only effectively police ourselves if we understand the implications of our actions. We simply cannot predict what someone else on this earth will try to do intentionally, and we cannot abet in the process of their carelessness. We can, however, put a moratorium on any funding that facilitates gain-of-function research. That is, at least, a reasonable first step.

I concluded at the end of *Fauci's Fiction* that society hasn't learned much from the COVID-19 pandemic. Most practitioners went back to testing and treating the way they did before they shuttered their doors and haven't adjusted to what the rest of us learned by being in the fight. In fact, patient care has gotten worse since the pandemic. Most people have gotten used to going to urgent cares. These facilities do not have a long-term record of you and cannot bill for follow-up visits. This means they don't think about the outcome and how your visit will affect you in the days down the road. They focus on the urgent need and address it without considering any follow up. In this instant gratification society, people have moved away from the general practitioner or primary care providers to speed things up and get immediate care. If we took the time to study what we did learn about the data, testing, and treatment, we would realize that we are still practicing in the 20th century and haven't made the leap into the 21st century!

We collected so much data through mass, forced testing during the pandemic that we can transform the way we look at respiratory pathogens and how we treat them. I didn't realize at the time that we were in the middle of a never-before-seen case study of viral and bacterial pathogens. We may never get that chance again during our lifetimes, and personally, I hope we never have to go through any of that again. However, it is a real shame that we can't study the data because of the censorship and cognitive distortion that exists about COVID-19. The same thing is happening with the COVID-19 vaccines. I don't use the word "vaccine" when discussing the mRNA shots that were administered because, as I've written previously, it's borderline malpractice to discuss a shot with an older population that may associate the word "vaccine" with that of an "inoculation". In *Fauci's Fiction*, I discussed that the definition of the word "vaccine" was changed during the pandemic to fit the narrative of the shots that were being administered. Most reasonable people associate the word "vaccine" with long-term immunity. If you consider a 120-day average antibody response "long-term", then you can feel free to call it a vaccine. My patients, who are a little bit older, may feel that this terminology can be vastly misleading.

While technically the terms "vaccination" and "inoculation" are interchangeable, a large segment of the population has become accustomed to expect that both will deliver long term or lifetime immunity. This is not the case with flu shots or Covid shots. In popular culture, flu shots were always referred to as just that, "flu shots". However, when Covid shots first appeared, they were referred to as "vaccines", and as the definition of the word "vaccine" was tweaked, flu shots are now often referred to as "flu vaccines".

This work is an extension of *Fauci's Fiction* as it tells the rest of the story of what our team and our teams of colleagues are seeing at ground level. We will talk about what the media and government aren't telling you and why the media outlets may not be picking up on the information. A lot of it has to do with the way it's reported, and there's more to that story than you may have anticipated. We will discuss the data that's publicly available, as well as the data that is being suppressed, or more importantly, ignored.

I know some keyboard warrior is going to look at the cover of this book and start screaming, "YOU'RE AN ANTI-VAXXER!" To which I'll say, "Funny, I mentioned you in the first chapter", in the hopes they might read it instead of making assumptions. The truth is, all "vaccines" are not the same. I examined that in detail in *Fauci's Fiction*, but the basics are that we've been using different types of technology for many years and those types were attenuated, viral vector, etc. They never included mRNA vaccines until we rushed them through approvals for the COVID-19 pandemic. Operation Warp Speed cut all the red tape to get these shots on the market, when it normally would have taken a minimum of four to five years.

To the person who hasn't read a word of the book but insists in screaming insults... I'll reiterate something I have always said. We didn't "not recommend" these shots because we thought there would be issues with them in the future, we didn't recommend these shots for two simple reasons. First, they didn't work! If you wanted a 120-day antibody response from these shots (like a flu shot), they may have made sense if the government recommended them before the seasonality of the virus, but they weren't doing that. Second, my patients simply didn't need them! Having not lost a single patient during the pandemic, coupled with the fact that all of them had already had COVID-19, a "vaccine" or essentially a "flu shot" wouldn't have made any difference.

You must remember that there was around a year of analyzing the data from positive COVID-19 patients before the shots existed. Out of my 19,000 patients and 4,000 positive cases, we didn't lose one patient. I only had four cases that we sent to the hospital for advanced medical care. So, if any of my more than 19,000 patients had asked, "Hey, do you think I need this shot?" The answer was a laughable NO! Why would I or any of my medical staff recommend untested technology for something that everyone was surviving without treatment? Most of these people had never even had a flu shot, but the campaign to advertise these Covid shots was so persuasive that most of the population fell for it.

When these Covid shots first became available, 75% of the American public got fully vaccinated. I can only hypothesize that most of our patient population was in the 25% that held off because they knew more than the rest of the world. It took quite a while for the masses to catch up to our early data and recommendations. As of this writing, only about 17% of the population has kept up with the boosters and is considered "fully vaccinated". Took them a while. I can usually spot these slow learners in every airport, still wearing masks. Apparently, they never read my first book, which discusses why we do NOT wear surgical masks for a virus. I wouldn't ask one of these people for directions to a gas station, never mind medical advice.

If you were one of those people who got your first shot and not your second, or two shots because you needed to travel or work, I get it... It's not your fault, and the powers that controlled the narrative at the time wouldn't let people like me speak to get the information out to you. It was more frustrating for me than it was for you, I promise. Seeing what we saw as early as March and April of 2020 and then again with the vaccines a year later, I was confident that the masses would have access to our information relatively soon. That never happened, and today, as I write this book, the censorship and misdirection continue. It still amazes me that, even four years after this virus first appeared, whoever is sensitive about getting this information out is still hard at work trying to keep it under wraps.

2

EVERYONE HAS A DIFFERENT TAKE

MY FRIEND LENNY TEXTED ME TODAY. He is 77 years old, a successful attorney, and passionate baseball coach. He told me a week ago that he had also come home from Yankee Fantasy Camp with Covid. Today, he wanted to update me on a potential player for our Yankee tournament series, but while he was texting me, he added that he "finally tested negative this past Saturday." I replied, "You really need to re-read my book." For the record, Lenny read my first book, and he should have been sufficiently educated on how testing works and how long a person is contagious. I reminded him by texting, "Do you go back to the doctor to ask when you are over the flu? Stop testing, it's inappropriate and unnecessary!"

Lenny then reminded me that he runs a baseball camp with 150 kids, and despite the science that he fully understands, those parents drive the narrative and still want to see a negative test before letting him back around their kids. So, it's the parents who need to read the book... It's frustrating because you can lead a horse to water, but you can't... well, you know the rest. What are we doing here, folks? We've essentially let the inmates run the asylum because they've outnumbered us, and we've lost control of the prison. There's a lot of people who still take trains to work, and all of them need to abide by the train schedule. They must pay attention, and be on time to catch the train, it's just how it works. We wouldn't hold the 7:10 train every day to accommodate the lazy passengers who got up late. If they read the schedule wrongly and didn't do their due diligence, then it's just too bad. We're not going to inconvenience everyone else who did! That's essentially what we have done during the past few years. While there are those of us who have educated ourselves on the "actual" science, the train is being held up for the rest of those who walk around using conjecture and assumptions to run their lives.

I don't know how to better metaphorically discuss what we are doing when it comes to Covid, testing, the shots, etc. We wore masks to make other people feel safe, even though, scientifically, they do not work for a virus. We succumbed to others' demands to get "vaccinated", even though the rhetoric that led to themselves getting vaccinated would have assured them that they "should have been protected" from anyone else who wasn't! To top it off, we still rush out to get COVID-19 tests to make others feel better and satisfy some ridiculous notions, all because of the lazy adults who can't learn or understand how science works in the first place. For the record, you can test positive for COVID-19 for up to 90 days on a PCR, but you aren't contagious after 14 days. The incubation period for Covid is three to five days, so once you develop symptoms, you are likely at around day four in the process. Once you add ten days of isolation, you are at fourteen days—and THAT'S THAT, no need to keep testing. That's for the parents who keep inconveniencing my good friend Lenny.

Also, to refresh, PCR testing works very differently than rapid antigen testing. Refer to the chapter on "How Testing Really Works" in *Fauci's Fiction* and you'll understand that you could be positive for a common cold on a rapid test. They don't look for co-infections, and you need a TON of viral material to trigger them positive, and that's *IF* you are even using them correctly. Throw those rapid antigen tests out already!

This reminds me of what our culture has become over the last few years... Everybody gets a trophy, there are no losers, etc. However, that rarely plays out in sports or in life. There are losers in life, and when we try to level the playing field by keeping down our stars, eventually, the game itself loses. We're doing the same thing when it comes to how we've responded to the pandemic. In this book, we are going to talk about what's in these shots, what they do, and some of the stories from patients and practitioners that you've never heard in the mainstream news. I've interviewed practitioners, scientists, and even embalmers to expose the real science behind these shots that were forced on the whole world. It's important to look at the data, and we will get there, but it's also important to breakdown why everyone may not be as receptive as you and me. It's important to understand the psychology at play and the attitudes the public has adopted regarding the narrative.

Everyone has a different take, and even if most people wind up eventually seeing the light, we have been forced to go along with the minority in an effort not to offend anyone for fear of being cancelled, shunned, or labeled an anti-vaxxer. All we've done by going along with the program is dumb down society even further... Don't try that at my workplace! I don't come to your job and make the same assumptions. However, lots of people did during this pandemic. Everybody has become an "expert" on communicable diseases, treatment, testing, and just about anything they have access to on the internet. For God's sake, stop making Lenny stick swabs up his nose because you don't understand how science works!

If you want to challenge me, tell me where you work, so I can come there and tell you that you're doing your job wrong. After a few hours, maybe you'll get the point... I probably have no experience in what you do for a living, but I'll pretend to, just to make my case! My team, the experts, the scientists who studied this every day with real data, do know a tad more than those "experts" on T.V. Those so-called "experts" have repeated the same CDC narrative from day one and don't have any practical experience. What we are going to explore in *Vaccine Fiction* is the hard truth, from the people who've done this for years and have no political bias. The data speaks for itself.

People seem to have a very myopic view about the "vaccines" and love to talk about their own personal experience because it somehow validates their opinions. My job as a researcher is to study and report the evidence, the numbers don't lie, and those numbers can paint a picture for you if you're willing to listen and put them in perspective. I didn't set out to study COVID-19 by choice, it just sort of happened. Fortuitously, we were the first company to start testing in our state. We had a head start on Covid before the masses even knew what it was, and like you, I was curious and eager to analyze the trends we saw to protect myself, my friends, and my family.

This myopic view people seem to cling to is a real problem. In an age where information is abundant and coming from all directions, most don't know what's real or what's just a flash in the pan. I've had many discussions with people who want to argue science based on their own personal experiences. Someone may have caught Covid and gotten very sick. In their minds, they may think that everyone experiences that same symptomatology. In our experience, which includes over 19,000 patients and over 4,000 positive cases, 85-90 percent of them were asymptomatic or mild. Someone may have gotten their "vaccinations" and felt completely fine. However, when you have a very large and diverse patient population, the narrative starts to shift.

The same would be correct for the person who had a severe adverse reaction to one of the shots, that just doesn't happen with every single person. We have had patients who have had adverse reactions right after their shot, or a medical condition that developed within a reasonable timeframe. When that does happen, it's very easy to see the cause and correlation. We've also seen patients develop issues much later. This is where it gets complicated to try and prove cause and correlation. However, when the metadata is put up against historical data, it's easy to see a clear connection to the rollout of the Covid shots.

Myopic views are dangerous because they convince the subject that there is no other alternative. For me, it's exhausting trying to explain all this to people who just want to argue with me because of a political narrative. Often, they'll have some visceral reaction to what they went through over the past few years due to Covid fatigue or some form of PTSD. I get it, it's frustrating! My biggest concern is always the credibility and reputation of myself and my staff. Please know that I always approach every conversation, writing, and interaction with credibility first and foremost in my mind. Once you say something inaccurate, it becomes the fruit of the poisonous tree, and everything else is tainted. We fastidious about ensuring our data is properly vetted before disseminating it to the public. My credibility is on the line, so I make sure we are 100 percent right before delivering that information to you.

The larger problem with these mRNA "vaccinations" is that people can develop an inflammatory response in an area of the body that's not immediately obvious to them. Many adverse reactions to vaccination are found in what's called "incidental findings". That's when a practitioner runs some tests and finds an illness incidentally, or beyond what they may have been looking for and intending to treat on that visit. I've heard too many stories of someone going into the hospital for what they think is a small and treatable issue only to find out that they have full-blown cancer that is now out of control.

What's even more dangerous is that people's political persuasion often leads them in a direction that is completely off-base. I've seen this on both sides and it's quite disturbing. Again, I'm a data guy, I call it like I see it. Don't get me wrong, the bias with COVID-19 is usually slanted more on one side than the other, but I think that comes down to the thought process mold and the fact that one side is more rooted in logic than the other. You can come to your own determination on that one...

The people on the left will argue that people on the right are anti-vax, which is a very broad statement and one I disagree with wholeheartedly. As previously mentioned, vaccines are not all the same. To call someone anti-vax because they didn't want to participate in an experiment with new mRNA technology would be blatantly false if that person has received other types of vaccinations. However, it seemed to be that the narrative mattered more than the reality of the data. Some people on the right got so adamant that Covid was "made up" that they associated anything to do with Covid as "fake". The truth lies somewhere in between, as it always does. Covid is very real, and there's a longer conversation to be had about where it came from. Further discussion can also be had on how it was funded, if it was part of "gain-of-function" research, and if there is culpability on the part of certain parties. After researching this for over four years of my life, I do believe there is...

People on the right will want to argue about PCR testing and its accuracy, and whether it should have been used in the first place. The stark reality is that we used PCR testing for many years before Covid even existed. When you use reputable labs that care about their own credibility, they do not deviate from the guidelines that they stake their reputations on. We didn't use Lab Corp and Quest. We used boutique labs that have been consistently reliable throughout many years of collaboration.

Sometimes I'll do an interview with a TV host who just wants to tear apart PCR testing for an hour. Keep in mind, our offices don't conduct PCR testing, the labs we work with do all the testing. And again, we've been using this type of testing for many years prior to the emergence of Covid. My full "RPP" or Respiratory Pathogen Panel has 31 different pathogens on it… That's 31 different coronaviruses, flus, viral pathogens, bacterial pathogens, and fungal pathogens. It's used to isolate which signal is in the sample and identify what the illness is. It also identifies how much viral load is in the patient. The people who want to tear this test apart say that if it's cycled up high enough, a person can find anything.

While this is technically true, any reputable lab won't go beyond 36 cycles. This is the cycle count used by both labs we worked with during the pandemic. People will then use the same argument to suggest that we would have a positive result in every single sample we collected. This is simply not true. You see, when the data is in front of you daily, and our office is matching that data with speaking to each patient and discussing their symptomatology, we would have been able to spot a trend that didn't make sense in practice.

In science, we look for something called repeatable data. For instance, if our office tested 100 people in a single day, we may have gotten 99 negative results and 1 positive result. I could repeat the process with the same grouping on the same day or the next day and get the exact same result for "exactly" the same people. This could be done over and over. This completely negates the arguments of the people who want to prove that PCR testing doesn't work and their hypothesis that we could find something on every single patient. I've had to repeat this for people who "think" they've gotten false positives. The confusion lies in the fact that most people who contract Covid do not get classic symptoms. The naysayers, according to their hypothesis, would have yielded 100 positive results regardless of symptomatology or repeat data. They just don't see the forest for the trees and have fixated on something that is now distracting them from the larger picture.

I hate having this PCR discussion with people who've read an article where "the creator of the technology says it should never be used to diagnose anything." The fact is, we have never in our lifetimes had that opportunity where we could essentially test a larger hypothesis. That is, what percentage of people infected by pathogens get classic symptoms? We found that about 85-90 percent of people infected were considered asymptomatic or had mild symptoms. Now, there is a little more to dive into here as well. You see, symptoms aren't always observable, sometimes they are only reportable. That means, when a patient is expecting to be "sick" or have what they believe to be classic symptoms, from what they've seen on the news, they expect a cough, a fever, or maybe even shortness of breath. Those symptoms are easily observable during a visit. However, the most common symptom from COVID-19 is a headache, followed by fatigue. This is important as I may be arguing with a patient who thinks they got a false positive because they don't have the "classic symptoms". They may come back for a retest only to get ANOTHER positive. Some get angry and want answers because it's negatively affecting their life or livelihood. When we sit down and talk about how Covid "really" works, it may take 20 minutes to explain the most common symptom is a headache. This is when they look up and say, "You know, I have been having some nasty headaches this week." This is something that's only reportable by a patient, it's not observable. My practitioners can't get inside their heads. They would all expect to be "sick" with the debilitating symptoms they had seen on television and what they had learned and come to expect with their limited knowledge up to that point. We have learned so much more since this experience, and we need to make sure that knowledge is understood by practitioners and patients moving forward.

For someone in my position, it's all about trying to combat everyone's own personal, preconceived and misinformed opinion. Keep in mind, I did this one person at a time before I put figurative pen to paper. It was frustrating to do this patient by patient during the pandemic, but it's even more frustrating now that I have published a book and still have to educate those who either haven't read it or are still stuck in some rabbit hole.

As a side note, the reason we had so many asymptomatic cases isn't a secret. Sick people, by definition, go to the doctor's office or maybe a hospital for care. Our office had sick people coming in, but most of the patients we attended to were from the weekly testing we conducted in facilities that forced their population to take the tests. Those consisted of police departments, assisted living facilities, and the countless amounts of travelers who needed a clean PCR test to travel on planes at the time. Some of those asymptomatic patients would later develop symptoms and some would not, but a lot of those symptoms just weren't being reported because they wouldn't call back to tell us they had experienced a massive headache and felt run down! I had to learn how to better explain "asymptomatic" so people would stop digging that rabbit hole even deeper. Our staff is very intelligent, and they had their finger on the pulse of this thing daily, for over three years. My staff and I see Covid very differently than the average person, and when you see it the way we do, the matrix is easy to navigate.

The broader point about the vaccines is that all these misconceptions and deviations distracted the masses. I used to discuss Covid one on one in my office with the belief that if we can just help one person at a time to understand this, we are making a difference. What I didn't realize at the time was that all this misinformation was spreading like wildfire, and we were getting behind the eight-ball. By the time the vaccines were released in 2021, a certain segment of the population was sternly one-sided, while others were also cemented in their thought process mold because the government and the media had handled this so poorly. Misinformation is one thing, but deliberately leaving out valuable information about the effectiveness of masks, the true mortality rate, how viruses transmit, and appropriate precautions—things that affect people's lives—is blatantly nefarious. Was it intentional? Did the government think we would all panic? If the government had just been transparent with the public, I think the adults in the room would have taken over and come to common-sense solutions. Instead, they treated the public like a room full of kindergarteners and hoped compliance would put everyone on the same page. What they were essentially doing was walking the public off a cliff, either forcibly or under the guise of voluntary compliance. This would have never happened if the truth about Covid or the "vaccines" was allowed to see the light of day.

As the vaccines began to roll out, people lined up and would figuratively knock each other over to be first to receive it. There existed another group of people who said NEVER EVER. There was another group, somewhere in the middle, that said, "Let me wait just a little bit and see what happens." Quite frankly, I wasn't in a rush to do anything besides handle the patient load we had at the time. We were still inundated with weekly testing at our contracted facilities and seeing an additional 100 to 200 patients in our physical offices daily. My NJ office never participated in the vaccine rollout, but we did distribute both the Moderna and Johnson and Johnson shots in our Key West office. In total, we didn't administer that many shots in our Florida office. That was partly because if a patient asked if we thought they "needed" it, our answer was a smirk with a head shake followed by an audible "NO". We hadn't lost any patients to date and weren't planning to. We had this under control, at least with our own patient population, but the number of vaccines we administered isn't the important metric. What really makes the difference in gauging the metrics was the fact that we had 19,000 patients, most of whom we got to know very well. We had years of horizontal data on these patients, and we even had separate antibody data on certain groups of them.

If a patient from one of our travel clinics decided to go off to a local pharmacy to get their shots, we would never know if they developed an adverse reaction unless they told us at one of our sites. However, we did see a lot of vaccinated patients for months and years after because they were still being forced to test weekly. We heard many stories of "breakthrough" cases and adverse reactions after the shots were administered. Some patients requested full antibody studies after "vaccination", which we could then measure against the previous antibody studies from natural infection. To date, I don't believe anyone else in the country has the same amount of horizontal data on such a vast number of patients as we do! When I think back on what we accomplished during that timeframe, I'm still amazed we were able to do it. However, I didn't know at the time that what we were doing was essentially a case study on the whole of the COVID-19 pandemic.

I'll reiterate from my previous book—I called every single positive patient from our daily list of positives. I called them every night, as soon as the results populated in our lab portal. To put that into perspective, this was a monumental task, not only to inform our patients the moment we had their results back, but to collect valuable data that nobody else in the country seemed to be collecting. If a patient went to a local pharmacy for a test, that patient was somehow notified of their results but wasn't questioned as to their symptomatology, how long it lasted, if it was followed up on, etc. We have some unique data in the industry that paints a very different picture of the pandemic.

This amount of data was pivotal in determining whether the Covid shots had any effect. We saw no appreciable difference in the ratios between sick and asymptomatic cases. In other words, the data didn't change. Before the vaccines were released, roughly 85 to 90 percent of our positive cases were asymptomatic or "not reporting symptoms", or didn't have the classic symptoms the patient expected to experience. After the vaccines were released, the numbers stayed the same, but the news outlets and the government narrative was such that if a patient was asymptomatic or "less severe" than they expected, it was, of course, thanks to the vaccine. This was a blatant lie, which we knew because we were looking at the numbers in real time. The government and any news outlet with a large audience never reported the early numbers. This means the narrative was completely made up! It was fabricated, it was misrepresented the entire time, likely to manipulate people into getting fully vaccinated. It took months before people realized that they could indeed catch Covid despite being fully vaccinated.

Everyone thought if they received a vaccine that their symptoms would be diminished. This wasn't the case. The data proves that the severity, or lack thereof, in the totality of the patients is exactly the same before the shots came out compared to after. It's a belief that people hold on to from their own myopic view of Covid. We now know, by looking at the real data, that those who were the sickest among us were either compromised or infected with one or multiple co-infections that added to their symptomatology. There are 31 different pathogens on a panel. If someone had Covid only (with no co-infection) and got sick, it was usually because they were compromised in another way, i.e., they were older, had asthma, cancer, etc. A person who was going to die in the next five years would not do well with any infection, and a younger person who only contracted Covid usually flaked it off unless they had a co-infection on the panel, i.e., flu, h flu, staph, etc. I once had a guy who had 4 infections at once… He was DEFINITELY sick with classic symptoms. The question I get the most after citing this is, "So, why were so many people dying of Covid early on?" Simply put, it was our lack of understanding what would work to treat them early on and using things like flu protocols which did not work for Covid. These protocols would actually exacerbate the virus! In addition, the novelty of the virus contributed to the miscommunication. By the time the vaccines were rolled out, the virus had already encircled the earth with global implications. By this time, most people had already experienced an initial reaction and developed B and T lymphocytes.

People had their own personal take depending on what their view was of their own illness or lack thereof. It often depended on the view of a loved one or what channel you were watching. Most if not all the news outlets got COVID-19 wrong in the early stages, but they were seeking opinions from experts who had shut the doors of their practices to avoid seeing infected patients and got talking points from the CDC. They should have consulted those of us who did this day in and day out. It would have changed the story dramatically. To those of you who tried, next time try harder. To those of you who perpetuated a narrative for ratings, karma is a dangerous thing. You contributed to a lot of mental and psychological anguish. You contributed to the degradation of society, and you have blood on your hands. You are just as culpable as the nefarious actors and medical "experts" that you shilled for. However, I've seen the misinformation spew on both sides, all for the sake of trying to prove a narrative. The truth is right in front of you if you are willing to look, and it doesn't come in the form of opinion. As Winston Churchill once said, "Facts are stubborn things!"

CENSORSHIP AND CLARIFICATION

EARLIER, I TOUCHED ON SOME CENSORSHIP issues, but I need you to understand exactly why you are not hearing vital information. I need you to understand that important information about Covid and the "vaccines" is deliberately being held from you. You have been misled by your own government.

Today was a very interesting day for me, and a day that brings some clarity to my own struggle to publish information on the pandemic. Recently released information verified some of the claims I have been making since my first book was released. The *New York Post* released a story where Congressman Jim Jordan, who is the chairman of the U.S. House Judiciary Committee, uncovered e-mails between President Joe Biden's White House and Amazon. The Biden Administration had specifically asked Amazon to suppress books that mention COVID-19 and the vaccines for fear that they may spread "misinformation". Amazon initially pushed back when asked to censor these types of books but eventually gave in. This explains why Amazon sent me three separate pieces of correspondence stating that I was not allowed to spend money to promote my book because of "current events". They said that I would be allowed to do so once this moratorium on these "current events" was lifted. Who decided this? The folks at Amazon never read my book. The people occupying the White House most definitely did not read my book. They never even read a review or synopsis of what the book is. They based this purely off an assumption from the cover and title! How many other authors have had their works shadow-banned at the direction of the White House?

Does Amazon have an algorithm or a team of reviewers who decide what is "misinformation" on COVID-19? This may not come as a shock to some of you, but for someone who is trying to market a book and get the truth out, it is unbelievably frustrating and harmful. It means a reader must type in the full title to find my books on Amazon. The algorithm won't suggest it if they are searching for keywords like "books on Covid" or "book on vaccines". The book will never surface in the search. Sometimes I do radio interviews that may last all of four minutes. It would be helpful if those listeners didn't need to write down the exact title or name of the author when looking for the book later. How much has this cost the authors, and WHY is that information being suppressed?

It makes you wonder how much of the information on vaccines is being hidden from you by all these big tech algorithms. If you really think about it, our entire world is big tech, from Amazon to Google to Facebook, Instagram, and all the other popular social media platforms. Most people now get their news from social media, and if the big search engines are censoring the truth, a person wouldn't be able to find the answers even if they were actively searching for them.

Today, I was on the phone with two different congressional offices and multiple attorneys to discuss the implications of this suppression of information and how it affected me. Will anything come of it? I'll let you know if things change before the book is finished, but I don't have much faith that it will. This is "par for the course" at this point, and I don't think anyone would want to implicate themselves in the process of coming clean. It may be time for some pressure. They are hoping that you have moved on and have banked on the fact that your rage and angst about all the draconian restrictions have calmed down.

Before I get into the vaccines and how Operation Warp Speed caused more harm than good, I'd like to mention something I didn't foresee when I wrote my first book. I recently did an interview on a show with a very large audience. The audience most likely votes the way I vote, but they tend to go down the conspiratorial rabbit hole, while I am a data guy who likes hard evidence. We spent the better part of the interview explaining PCR testing. I've found myself having to do this more often as there were numerous stories making the rounds that the validity of these tests was in question. It seems that a lot of these people have gravitated towards these types of stories and latched onto them to say "gotcha". I thought we had a great interview, and the host couldn't have been nicer. Now, I know if I had simply asked any of his audience, "How many people did *you* test and treat during covid?" the answer would be zero, unless they were referencing their own myopic view of themselves or someone they know. It's highly likely that they did not test over 19,000 patients over 44,000 times and look at 44,000 reports, compare the data, speak to each patient about symptomatology, and record that data, but I could be wrong! Yet, I was met with a barrage of comments from the interview such as:

"Something is fake about this guy."

"He's obviously trying to cover his tracks."

"How could they find Covid on a PCR if the virus was never isolated?"

"Even the inventor of PCR testing said you can't use it to diagnose, and he died."

"He's part of the conspiracy and an obvious plant."

You get the idea. But there were also plenty of choice words used in the more than 80 comments I looked at before I had to stop reading them. Hey look, if you have a bias against PRC testing, I can't stop you from having that bias because if you believe it, it must be true! I'm pretty sure you haven't ever used the test, and I'm pretty sure you don't consult an immunologist on CT value and how the testing works. My point is, everyone in his audience, well almost everyone, couldn't see the forest for the trees because they had gotten stuck on this one myth. Now I've explained how testing works, which I went over extensively in *Fauci's Fiction*, I'll also stipulate that if any of these naysayers want to come to my office for one day and look at how things work, study the data, and analyze the ins and outs of what we do, it would make them look very foolish for perpetuating this nonsense.

I didn't enter the sphere of Covid testing with an agenda. A reputable scientist will present a hypothesis and formulate a valid or null hypothesis upon analyzing the data. Naysayers look for anything to disprove PCR testing, and therefore, by that logic, covid isn't real and we've all been had. Well, we have all been had but for very different reasons. PCR testing was at the root of explaining that, and not for the reasons the naysayers think. It was PCR testing in abundance that gave us true numbers as to the spread. It allowed us to see how many mild cases vs severe cases of Covid were in existence, and it allowed us to prove that medicine had been mismanaged for all the years leading up to Covid. We can learn a lot if we analyze the data we derived during this period, but the naysayers need to hear the full story.

I have no horse in this race except my credibility and the health of our patients. If I saw for even one second that PCR testing was a bogus resource, we would have stopped using it to protect our credibility and patients. The fact remains that PCR testing, when done correctly, is the only way to diagnose COVID-19. Any reputable scientist will tell you so, and it's mostly because of the inaccuracy and sensitivity of antigen testing. I didn't think I would hear this argument when I released *Fauci's Fiction*, but I've heard it enough times now that I feel the need to clarify a few things. The data makes more sense when you see it day in and day out. It almost paints a picture like a matrix. You can spot the trends and see where it's all headed. Like the fact that most people coming in at very high CT values did not develop classic symptoms, which makes sense. They didn't have a high viral load, and the replication didn't inhibit the overall health of the patient. We ran full panels on sick patients, which taught us that most people with classic symptoms had co-infections. This is something that wasn't being looked at by other clinicians or quick testing sites. PCR testing also helped validate positive rapid antigen tests, where roughly 98 percent of the time a positive rapid antigen would then come back positive on a PCR test. However, one cannot confirm Covid on a rapid antigen test because of the instances of positives that would be triggered by other coronaviruses.

It's funny to me that everyone in the world has become an "expert" on virology, epidemiology, and immunology. I'm at least aware enough to know that I don't know everything, but I can learn from the best and learn something new every day if my mind isn't closed off to accepting new knowledge. I wanted to make that clear because we are going down another road with the vaccines, but sometimes other issues become sticking points for readers, and they then invalidate anything associated with the work. Now, I know, when you're explaining, you're losing, but I think it's worthwhile to touch on this as it is the basis for most of the data we derived from the pandemic.

If you look hard enough at the data, it backs up the naysayers' larger claims that Covid wasn't that big of a deal when it comes to health concerns, they just need to get out of their own way sometimes!

Sometimes I wonder if the censorship war is all planned. These powers have done an extensive job of censoring the information we garnered during the pandemic. This wasn't just me; it was a lot of other reputable practitioners and scientists as well. Do they also have a hand in burying the truth about the pandemic by planting information to make sure both sides sound irrelevant? The older and less experienced me would have said, nah... that's too farfetched. The new and more experienced me would say, it's probably more than plausible at this point. I'm quite sure what you are about to hear regarding the vaccines may sound a little farfetched too, but I will make a friendly wager with you that what you hear now, you will DEFINITELY hear at some point in the future, as the truth tends to leak out, even in small doses.

The fact is, as I researched some of the data for this book, at certain points, part of me recoiled. I asked myself, "Do I really want to risk my reputation by including this in the book?" However, as the months went on, and I heard some of this data being backed up by other scientists, practitioners, and independent researchers, I started to feel more confident about the book but scared shitless about the reality of what had just happened in the world. As the stories of people dying suddenly appeared daily, the question then became, "Do you think it was related to the vaccine?" For example, recent stories of rare cancers are abundant and coming out of every corner of the world. Most of these cancers have a rapid onset, and many are full-blown before a patient even realizes they are sick. These stories may wake you up a bit if you aren't being led down a road that doesn't have access to that information. "Nothing to see here!"

Today, as I write this, I learned that my friend Marilyn passed away. I mentioned her and her husband Phil in *Fauci's Fiction*, and she is probably the only person that will get a second mention in this book besides her husband and my parents. She had been battling lung cancer over the past few years, but just three months ago, her scans were clear. They sold their house in New Jersey where they had lived for over 20 years and decided to move to Florida full-time. It was an arduous process to sell their home, not because of a bidding war but because of the memories and sheer number of possessions they had to go through before they could settle in another state. My family and I have had many Thanksgivings and Christmas dinners over at their New Jersey home, and when I bought my new home, it happened to be about 0.4 miles from where they resided. It was also tough on myself and my family when they decided to move a thousand miles away, nonetheless, we knew we would see them in their new digs in sunny Florida.

I'm torn as I write this because I want to make a point without sounding coy. I had warned Marilyn and Phil about the dangers we were seeing in the Covid shots. I had repeatedly told them, much like I had told my father before he passed, that the risk versus reward with these shots was not worth it. In the months leading up to her passing, we had discussed the amounts of rare and aggressive cancers we were seeing in practice from all around the world and how the staggering numbers in the amount increased directly following the mass vaccination of the entire populace. I took a trip down to Florida to see her just two short weeks ago. When I called to tell her I was coming, she and I spoke for a bit. She teared up telling me what she was feeling and said, "Michael, I don't know how this happened, my scans were completely clear three months ago, and now this." I paused for a few seconds and said to her, "We have been seeing a lot of this lately." She then took a few seconds before responding, "Yeah, I know, you should probably write another book about it!"

When I went to visit, knowing it may be the last time we were to see each other on this earth, we laughed, we cried, and we were optimistic. She mentioned three weddings that she had to attend in the following few months and how determined she was to make it to them. She told me that she was going to fight and beat this, but she knew all too well that she didn't have much time left. My wife and stepson were able to FaceTime with her. They were eager to speak with her, and I think it helped them more than Marilyn. This news was devastating for them as well, but they didn't want to make her feel uncomfortable by calling on days when she wasn't feeling her best. The time for them to say their last words to her was during this call. After a few hours, we said our goodbyes and said that we loved each other. I gave Phil a hug and turned one last time to say to Marilyn, "I will talk to you soon," which she then repeated with a big smile, "YES, I will talk to you soon!" Alas, just two short weeks later, she was gone.

I write this for two reasons. First, to immortalize a great woman, a wonderful mother, grandmother, and friend. Marilyn was a philanthropist who helped so many people in her lifetime. She didn't have a negative bone in her body and was always the first to help someone less fortunate. She was constantly inviting people over for a meal and fed half her block on most days. Marilyn was an optimist and was the first to congratulate you with a smile or offer words of encouragement when things looked darkest. I distinctly remember calling her only a year before she passed to tell her my father had died. She immediately broke down sobbing because of her love for him and just the fact that she was emotionally connected to the world and my family.

Secondly, I write this because, as sad as I am today, this news made me angry. Marilyn had her health problems, and she didn't take care of herself the way she should have, but I've seen this one too many times now. I've heard of too many cases of cancer coming on with a vengeance over the last few years. Could her death have been preventable? Every time a sudden death occurs these days, everyone in my circle asks, "Were they vaccinated?" When a young athlete has a heart attack or drops dead on the basketball court or gridiron, that's usually the first question that comes up, and quickly!

I'm angry because we were always ahead of the curve and our fingers were on the pulse of Covid, testing, the shots etc. My staff and I knew there would be long-term side effects to these shots and tried to tell anyone within earshot of what we were seeing, but it would always fall on deaf ears. The media and the government narrative drowned us out at every turn. If anyone is culpable for the uptick in sudden deaths and huge increase in cancer cases, it's the media just as much as the government. I could have told Marilyn until I was blue in the face that she didn't need or even want those shots, but the media narrative was so powerful, I looked like a tiny fish in a big pond, even though we had more horizontal data than anyone on the planet.

In Marilyn's case, we will never really know. Nobody will put pen to paper and try to figure out if her cancer was caused by those mRNA shots. All I can tell you is exactly what I told her, "We've been seeing this a lot lately." I can type about it until my fingers fall off, but once you start to see some of these charts and the way they compare to the last 30 years of data, you may start to see the same trends that I see every day. It's one thing to talk about it and tell anecdotal stories, but it's another to see the information right in front of your face. You'll see for yourself just how shocking this data is in the upcoming chapters.

In my last book, I didn't draw any conclusions, I just presented the data, figuring the reader was smart enough to figure it out. In some instances, just showing your data works, but unfortunately, most people need it spelled out to them. They don't want to have to do any work to get to the bottom of the story, they just want it told to them. In this book, I may come to more conclusions because the approach of just giving people the data obviously hasn't made a large enough impact. In Marilyn's case, she may be alive today if she had taken what I was saying a little more seriously than she did while this was all being rolled out.

When I first told my wife Kelly about Marilyn's diagnosis, she got quiet and visibly upset. She knew that the last set of treatments she went through was tough, and somehow, she overcame it. This time, Kelly felt it would be different. Kelly has worked in medicine for 15 years and is a wonderful family nurse practitioner. Before becoming an APRN, she worked in trauma, the float pool, and just about anywhere the hospital needed help. She was a preceptor for new nurses and has been nominated and won many prestigious awards over the course of her career. She is great at what she does and can usually figure out what the best and brightest can't because of her years of experience and dedication she puts into her craft.

After Kelly got a little quiet and upset, she just blurted out, "It's those fucking shots again!" This time, I reeled her back in for a second and said, "Well, you can't know that for sure, she did have her health problems all these years." It wasn't until Kelly looked at me and said, "But it's happening everywhere, it's too obvious at this point." That's when I realized I was trying to be too subtle about what I'd seen. I needed to be more "matter of fact." I'm not sure how many shots Marilyn got throughout the pandemic, but I do blame her doctors, the media, and the government for playing a part in her death. These abundances of cancers we are seeing with rapid onset match exactly what Marilyn had. Just a year ago, we were celebrating that she had beaten her previous onset of cancer and talking about our futures and what life had in store for all of us. Now we are trying to console her husband but also comparing her situation with the thousands of other similar instances we've seen since the shots rolled out in 2021.

There are no coincidences in life, and this set of circumstances mimics what we are seeing worldwide. I'm angry because this probably could have been prevented. I'm angry at myself for not speaking louder, for not making the point clearer that getting those shots was the single most irresponsible thing I have ever seen in my career. There was no need for it, and they didn't work. Somehow, I feel partly responsible as the first company to test for and treat COVID-19 and one of the first with horizontal data related to those shots. I can't turn back the clock, but maybe, just maybe, somebody will read this and think twice before rushing out for another "booster". It's too late for Marilyn and truthfully, we'll never really know, but my suspicions are based on more than just conjecture.

Anecdotal stories and family and friends aside, the human species is having a significant reaction to something we did between the years 2021 and the present day. What did we do differently? Well, the onset of Covid itself is a factor, but after surviving COVID-19 and the draconian measures that came along with it, a lot of my patients had some serious reactions and complications from the shots. Some of them flat out didn't survive.

I wrote in my first book about an assisted living facility where we tested weekly. After they had a few initial deaths due to Covid, the remaining population did well during the phase after Covid started and until the shots were readily available. As seniors who were "most vulnerable", they were prioritized to be given shots before anyone else. Out of roughly 60 of them who received the shots, 6 of them had serious complications, 3 died, and 3 had strokes within 2 weeks of the shots being administered. That's 10 percent of the patient population, for those of you who are counting.

The New Jersey state mandate required these facilities to use PCR testing, but now allows them to use rapid antigen tests to keep in compliance. We have not been in contact with the facility since, and have no idea as to the long-term effects those shots may have had on their remaining patient population. I'll add, the decision by the state to allow rapid antigen tests has to rank up there with one of the most ridiculous things I've ever seen by a government entity. I'm not sure who is advising these folks, but they sure don't have a clue. If you understand how testing works (explained in-depth in Chapter 9 of *Fauci's Fiction*), you'd know that you CANNOT diagnose Covid on an antigen test and the likelihood that you get a false negative is extremely high when someone's CT value is low. It puts the "most vulnerable" population at risk. However, we knew as early as April 2020 that the mortality rate would be close to that of the seasonal flu. It's quite obvious that the State of New Jersey and any other state mandating this type of testing is purely putting on a show.

Most of the mitigation didn't work in the first place. The fact that these government entities put these poor seniors through absolute hell, making them shove swabs up their noses every week, is proof that the government doesn't care about you. They only care about optics. When we weren't sure what was happening around us, testing was the ONLY way to find out. However, once we had a large enough sample size, which only took about two months, the government should have re-evaluated and put on the brakes. They didn't, and that spells manipulation to anyone who can put two and two together. I didn't mention any political narratives in *Fauci's Fiction*, but if you ask me if I thought something nefarious was going on, you'd have to lack brain cells and basic common sense to think otherwise.

So why don't you hear about these cases? Why don't you hear about this abundance of cancer and rapid onset, especially in young people? Well, it has to do with the way data gets reported and where it gets reported to! The story is only as good as the person doing the research, but if the research isn't available, how could you put it on the 6 O'clock news? If the data exists, but doesn't exist under the light of day, it makes it very difficult for anyone who's curious to even cite a case. You may hear things here and there. You may talk to people who tell you that there's "something" going on, but where can one go to pull records and compare notes? Where can you find the definitive source of vaccine related injuries and deaths? Have you heard of VAERS?

4

WHAT IS VAERS AND HOW DOES IT WORK?

VAERS, which stands for Vaccine Adverse Events Reporting System, was created in 1990 by the Centers for Disease Control and Prevention (CDC) and the United States Food and Drug Administration (FDA). VAERS was set up to track vaccine adverse reactions and be an early warning system for vaccine safety. It allows just about anyone to report into the system, including medical personnel, pharmaceutical companies, and even the patients themselves. While the CDC cites VAERS as having a "proven track record of successfully helping to identify safety issues", there are inherent problems with the reliability of the data in the system. Recording data alone does not correlate a reported vaccine adverse event with a medical issue. In other words, just because a patient reports an adverse event or medical issue, the system does not correlate the two. Further investigating needs to be done to determine whether the vaccine is linked to the medical event.

My interest in VAERS isn't to undercut the system or to criticize how and why it was set up. In fact, I think the intention behind VAERS was and is a good one. However, what's important to note here, and coming from an analyst, is that the data doesn't lie unless someone is pulling data from a skewed source. To add some context here, you'd have to look at the way Covid numbers were reported in the beginning stages, compare that to the present, and then compare that to how the VAERS system works. When the pandemic started, PCR was the only testing available as a rapid antigen test did not yet exist. Also, the COVID-19 emergency order didn't exist. However, CLIA laboratories are required by law to report infectious diseases to the states in which the test was conducted. In other words, in the beginning, a patient needed to exhibit symptoms or have a medical necessity to qualify for a test. If that patient came back positive for Covid, the lab would report those numbers to the appropriate state. Once the CARES Act was established and an emergency order was put in place, anyone at any time could get a COVID-19 test regardless of symptomatology or medical necessity. What we found, once this emergency order was established and the public panic ensued to rush out for a test, was that EVERYONE HAD COVID. Okay, well not everyone, but more people than you'd think. We learned a lot through this exercise of mass testing that we can use to study medicine as we progress into the future.

When we saw such a high number of cases with patients with very mild symptoms, we learned that not everyone got terribly sick from Covid. Think about it, in the past, you would only run out to get a test at a practitioner's office if you had classic symptoms like a cough, fever, or shortness of breath. In this instance, we had people rushing out to get tests out of pure panic and fear. The point here is that the COVID-19 numbers that were coming into the CDC and related agencies were relatively accurate because those labs were required to report by law and because we were using very sensitive and accurate testing measures. When we get into analyzing the vaccine rollout, one of the most important things we fail to discuss in the public forum is the number of people who were asymptomatic or had mild symptoms and recovered quickly. I don't think the masses would have rushed out to get experimental vaccines if they knew that the survival rate was reportedly 99.98% without any medical treatment whatsoever. This data set was relatively accurate, but the government and media refused to analyze it in totality. However, they did exploit the sheer volume of case load. The advent of the rapid test forced those "reported" numbers to go down artificially. Furthermore, the expiration of the emergency order and CARES Act, which now requires patients to have a symptom like a cough, a fever, or shortness of breath, means most patients with a medical necessity don't even qualify to get a test. That means, the cases are still out there, but we will never know about them because we are not constantly testing everyone anymore. I hope that makes sense. Basically, the only ones who qualify are those with classic symptomatology. However, most cases, in our experience, do not have classic symptomatology... SO BASICALLY, ALL THOSE CASES ARE STILL OUT THERE BUT WILL NEVER BE REPORTED! It does NOT mean that the numbers are down, and it does NOT mean that the vaccines worked. It's all artificial!

Let's look at how this works with the VAERS system. Federal law states that a practitioner must report a vaccine adverse reaction to the VAERS system. However, many practitioners do not use VAERS, and some don't even know the system exists. The numbers in VAERS don't even come close to reported COVID-19 cases, even with the skew in data we've come to see after rapid testing and emergency orders were rescinded.

In speaking with a practitioner, it becomes glaringly obvious as to why most vaccine related injuries go unreported. I had a very long interview with one such practitioner who was fired from her job because she decided to follow the law and do what was right. She gave me a lot of insight into how VAERS works in practice and why some of this data may not be making it into the system. To protect her identity, let's just call her Molly. Molly had been working for a mid-size hospital system as a mid-level practitioner, treating patients for many years before the pandemic began. Like most practitioners and nurses I have interviewed, when Covid happened, they rolled up their sleeves and put their faith in their bosses, their colleagues, and the government, including the CDC. It wasn't until a few months into the COVID-19 pandemic that these health care professionals started seeing inaccuracies in what they were being told by the government and media narrative. What they were seeing was stark and right in front of their eyes. The highlight reel on television didn't always match the box score of the actual game, nonetheless, these practitioners kept showing up for work every day!

You've got to remember, in this timeline of the pandemic, the vaccines didn't roll out until late 2021. Practitioners had been seeing some weird stuff when it came to Covid in general. They were all waiting with bated breath to see what the new mRNA technology vaccines would produce. I think most of the health care community had high hopes for these vaccines, and early data from the pharmaceutical companies also looked promising, citing 77 to 95 percent efficacy rates. If there were to be any side effects, we were unaware, but we were always cautious going into uncharted territory. mRNA technology had never been used before on a mass scale, but an attenuated vaccine would take much longer to produce. If the world was going to cut Covid off at its knees, we needed something fast and effective, at least that was the thought in the public at large and among the scientific community.

My offices and my staff had given many vaccinations over the course of their careers and much of what I knew of the procedures for vaccinations was standard. There are vaccine schedules that outline when a particular vaccination is recommended and for what age group. Any patient receiving a vaccination would then sit in an exam or waiting room after receiving their dose to make sure they did not have an adverse reaction or anaphylaxis. From all the vaccinations I've ever observed, I don't recall anyone ever having a medical emergency, except for a few patients whose blood pressure tanked, and our office needed to call 911 because one patient had an anxiety attack. This happens more often than you think, but I've personally never seen a reaction from a shot being administered directly. I polled dozens of other practitioners to ask them if they'd ever reported anything to the VAERS system, and the answer was always "no!" Most of the time, they didn't know what I was talking about because they had never heard of it in the first place. It was difficult to believe that none of them knew of VAERS considering the law in place to mandate reporting. Mostly, if a patient gets through that fifteen-minute window after receiving a shot, the patient is sent on their way and that's the end of it!

If a patient develops an issue after those fifteen minutes are up, the likelihood that the incident makes it into VAERS is low. Also, the further away an issue develops outside that window, the less likely it is to be determined in any way related to the vaccine. One would think that an open reporting system would have its benefits, but there are a few problems with the system even before we get to the CDC investigation into each incident. A few of the obvious reasons the system is flawed are:

1. Lack of knowledge of the VAERS system.
2. Proper training in using VAERS.
3. Proper enforcement.
4. Cognitive dissonance or distortion.

As I mentioned earlier, many of my staff had not heard of the VAERS system until Covid made it a household name, and even if they had heard of it, they had never used it or were never properly trained in how to do so. On top of that, they didn't know it was established law that they had to report any issues into the system. However, the larger issue would be cognitive dissonance or distortion. If a patient developed an issue that seemed to correlate with a shot being given, the further outside the fifteen-minute window they had for anaphylaxis, the further away they got from being a data point that you would ever hear about! To emphasize, if the reaction never makes it into the VAERS system, it's as if the event doesn't exist because the data doesn't exist.

No practitioner wants to admit that their recommendations caused an issue, no matter how much protection they had from the government. A lot of these general practitioners have had some of their patients in their practice for many years. They are mostly family doctors, and trust is of the utmost importance between the practitioner and the patient. If a patient came to them and asked the doc, "Do I need this shot?", these practitioners were often quick to give them an answer and looked towards the CDC. When their patient fit the recommended criteria, the practitioner, without having any experience with said shots, would give a scripted answer so they would appear to know what the hell they were talking about!

The best answer should have been an honest one that included the words, "I don't know." Hell, the CDC didn't have any long-term data, but these doctors steered their patients down a path that they can no longer come back from. Why, because they wanted to "appear" smart. You know what they say about the word assume, right? Not only did they make themselves and the entire industry look ridiculous, but they may also have been the cause for some of these incidents that ARE or ARE NOT being reported. For the patient who still trusts these practitioners' opinions, you may have discussed your adverse reaction case with the same person who was adamant about you getting that shot. Do you really think they would ever want to admit they took you down the wrong path? It's too bad most patients don't know that they can report these cases themselves. However, how often is a case reported to a practitioner's office and the patient assumes that the office will do the reporting, yet nothing is ever done? The system is just not set up as seamlessly as it is for laboratory reporting, so most of the numbers don't ever make it into VAERS.

This is where Molly comes in... Molly was kind of like the rest of us in that she didn't know much about the VAERS system until Covid appeared. She worked as a hospitalist in her system and was very well respected. She had won multiple awards throughout her career and had the trust and respect of her colleagues. Molly was just like the rest of us at the beginning of the pandemic, she was trepidatious, but eager to help kick this thing's ass because that's who she is, a fighter and an advocate for her patients. I have always admired people like Molly, she is well respected because she's earned it, and at the same time, she's always doing right by everyone else. She was sacrificing herself and her advancement along the way because her concern for others outweighed any self-centered notion she may have had for her own wellbeing. She was and is a true hero in this story—although sometimes the hero gets cast as the antagonist in the plot for a bit until the audience realizes the truth behind the narrative and the story starts to become clearer. As I've said in previous writings, these are the folks that get burned at the stake for declaring the earth is round and going against the grain. They are right, but nobody else can see it at the time, and when the masses catch up, it's too little too late.

When the vaccines rolled out across the country, Molly was working as a mid-level provider at her hospital. She started to hear stories of patients who were coming in with "adverse reactions" to what was "most likely" a recent vaccination. She started doing some research and looked for some avenues to report these instances. This is where she learned about the VAERS system. What she found was that VAERS had been in existence for quite some time and there was a process and procedure set up to report exactly that, any vaccination related reaction. She also discovered that practitioners were legally obliged to report such instances into this system. She had never done this before, and she started to ask questions of her colleagues.

When Molly asked around her hospital system if anyone had any experience with this reporting system or if any of her colleagues had ever used it, the answer she got was a resounding NO, just like when I had asked those same questions. She was then left to her own devices to figure out a method to the madness. Molly discovered that the process for reporting to VAERS can be time-consuming and cumbersome. It can take as long as 30 minutes to navigate the system to log an adverse reaction. The practitioner would need a lot of patient data as well as the lot numbers of each vaccine given to each patient. If you remember, during the pandemic, a lot of people were running off to their local CVS or Walgreens to obtain a shot. The practitioner would have to take the time to call each of those places to obtain lot numbers and dates of vaccination. Oh, and at any time, if the system glitched during this process, or the internet lost connectivity, or there was a power failure, the person doing the data entry would then have to start the process all over again. To put it mildly, it was a royal pain in the ass for a practitioner to take time out of their busy day even to report one patient into VAERS, and nobody wanted to do it.

On top of the time constraints of reporting a case to VAERS, the overwhelming cognitive distortion that is associated with a practitioner even wanting to report on something that they themselves recommended skews the reliability of VAERS before we even get any deeper into this conversation. Molly stepped up at the time, thinking she was doing her best to advocate for those patients coming in with issues and for the other practitioners who knew Molly was onto something. Most of the other providers knew that Molly had taken the lead and asked her if she would then take on the task of putting their patients into VAERS for them if they had anyone come back who was questionable. She took it upon herself to become the point person in her hospital system to do just that.

Molly wanted to make sure that this data entry was done correctly and that any one of the system's patients who had a concern had an outlet for being heard. Although the VAERS system was set up with good intentions, when you report a case, it doesn't automatically become a statistic. It is a way for agencies and the CDC to track and see if there are any potential problems with new vaccines, specific lot numbers, etc., and have some checks and balances along the way. What better way to track patient data than directly from the practitioners who would notice first line issues. It's a very quick way to recognize issues and deal with them at lightning speed. When the CDC can spot trends, it helps regulate the whole industry and cut off any major issues before spreading like wildfire. The problem here was, nobody had ever been trained in how to do this, what the system was, and what it was intended for. It took the onset of Covid for most practitioners to utter the term VAERS and find out what it was. Even now, most people have never logged into the system to report an anomaly, but they mention it in passing as a place where data is collected and used as a reference.

The system was set up so that anyone, not just a practitioner, could report into it. Even the patients themselves could do it! It wasn't set up to be a dirty word or a reference point for later clarification. It was set up to be easy to use, at least in the creators' minds, and to help the government spot trends and issues as an early warning measure before mass chaos broke out. The problem was, nobody knew it even existed! So here we are in the middle of a worldwide pandemic, people's lives are stunted, normalcy is on hold, and Molly is trying to notify the entirety of her hospital system that this "thing" exists to help mitigate some of the issues that are coming through the door. "I got this," she said, "I'm happy to learn the system, put the cases in, and be the point person in our system to make this happen." So, that's what she did, logging her own patients and even happily helping other practitioners in her hospital system by logging their patients at their request. Molly was becoming an expert at doing the work and logging the data. The fact is, nobody else in her orbit even wanted to touch it because it was too time-consuming.

This went on for about 150 cases before Molly's superiors started to get weary of the entire practice. Molly had been trying to get the other practitioners trained in the aspects of reporting, it was, after all, the law, and the hospital system seemed to be unaware of the law or of the importance of logging these cases. In Molly's words, "in their eyes, it was a waste of time." They told her that nationally, there didn't seem to be many issues with these shots, and they didn't want to cause "vaccine hesitancy". Wow, so I guess, if everyone lies, fails to report the cases, we can get more people "vaccinated" and worry about any ramifications later? That was exactly why VAERS was set up in the first place! This was to be the warning system, but someone pulled the plug out of it so the alarm would never sound. It's like setting up a tsunami warning system but unplugging it during the earthquake because they didn't want to cause panic about a tsunami that "could" come! The data was being swept under the rug. If the news didn't cover it, does that mean it never really happened?

After a few conversations with her superiors, Molly was eventually let go—that's a nice way of saying she was fired from her hospital system because her efforts to do the right thing and follow the letter of the law didn't align with the objectives of her hospital's management. Do you want to know what happened in her hospital system once Molly stopped reporting cases? You guessed it, nothing was entered into VAERS unless a patient took it upon themselves to figure out the cumbersome system. Imagine if you go to the police station to file a report, but the cops are all new and don't know how to log in to file a report. Imagine the FBI coming in five years later to compile crime data for your city but your case and countless others never made it into the system. The crime data would be skewed, but nobody would ever know about it. The data only makes it into the mainstream if it's recorded. You may think you live in one of the safest communities in the country, but the data never made it to its endpoint. In the case of Molly and her hospital system, what her superiors were doing and most likely are still doing is outright negligence.

Cognitive distortion comes to mind again, especially in this scenario because COVID-19 and the shots were so politicized. Everyone wants to be on a side, whether they are virtue signaling and wearing a mask, or they blatantly ignore data and any information that is counter to their narrative or the narrative they bought into and fought so hard to preserve. That's not how science evolves. In fact, science evolves by spurring rigorous debate where hypotheses are tested and retested. The "science" evolves when all the facts can be observed and weighed. When the facts are hidden from you or just simply ignored and discounted because it doesn't match the narrative of the day, society loses, and we don't grow. In fact, we regress!

Molly is now taking a break from medicine, but realistically, she's needed now more than ever. I can't blame her for wanting to distance herself from a hospital system that put lives at risk and systematically worked to hide the truth of these shots from the public. However, without people like Molly, the world would never know the arrogance and negligence of how some of these systems are run. It is my opinion that much of the world will never know the truth about Covid and the damage these shots have caused because most people responsible for compiling and analyzing the data are already tainted with a bias.

Administrators wanted to take the path of least resistance, in some cases because Medicare (the largest payer) indicated that they would not pay hospitals if their staff wasn't "vaccinated", or they were making it very hard on their patient population to do business with the system if they weren't also "vaccinated". In other words, the hospital bought into this nonsense hook, line, and sinker, and for them to go back on their word now after such a hard push would make them look, well... pretty damn stupid, and everybody wants to save face and not look like a complete idiot. The hard truth is, when the majority of the practitioners finally catches up to people like Molly, they will look pretty stupid—but they'll never admit it! They'll spin it with comments like, "Well, we just didn't know back then." They'll say things like, "We were doing the best we could." But we did know, and they were summarily ignorant. Molly knew, she tried to tell people, they just didn't care enough about their patients to push their own political bias out of the way!

5

WHAT WE KNEW ABOUT VACCINES BEFORE COVID

The History of Vaccine Development

Before COVID-19, vaccines were regarded as one of the greatest medical innovations in human history. Their development has dramatically reduced the prevalence of deadly diseases, saved millions of lives, and continued to play a crucial role in public health. From the early days of smallpox variolation to modern mRNA vaccines for COVID-19, the history of vaccine development is a tale of scientific discovery, innovation, and perseverance.

Early Beginnings: Variolation and the Fight Against Smallpox

The first known attempt at immunization, though rudimentary by today's standards, occurred in ancient China around the 10th century. People practiced a technique called variolation, where material from smallpox sores was either inhaled or rubbed into small cuts on the skin. The goal was to induce a mild form of the disease, which would then provide immunity against more severe cases of smallpox.

Variolation was also practiced in Africa and the Middle East. It wasn't until the early 18th century, however, that the technique was introduced to Europe, where it gained significant attention. Lady Mary Wortley Montagu, the wife of the British ambassador to the Ottoman Empire, observed the practice in Constantinople (modern-day Istanbul) and, upon her return to England, advocated for its use.

While variolation did reduce mortality from smallpox, it was not without risks. Sometimes, the procedure led to full-blown smallpox infections, which could be fatal. Additionally, because the technique used a live smallpox virus, it had the potential to spread the disease to others.

Edward Jenner and the Birth of Vaccination

The turning point in vaccine history came in 1796 with Edward Jenner, an English physician who is often credited as the father of modern immunology. Jenner noticed that milkmaids who contracted cowpox, a much milder disease, seemed immune to smallpox. Based on this observation, he hypothesized that exposure to cowpox could protect against smallpox.

To test his theory, Jenner took material from a cowpox sore on a milkmaid's hand and inoculated it to an eight-year-old boy named James Phipps. Several weeks later, Jenner exposed the boy to smallpox, but he did not develop the disease. Jenner's experiment was a success, and this technique became known as "vaccination," derived from the Latin word "vacca" for cow.

Jenner's discovery laid the foundation for the development of future vaccines. Although his methods were crude by modern standards, they were revolutionary for their time. His work also prompted other scientists to explore immunization, and by the mid-1800s, vaccination had become a widespread practice in Europe and North America.

The Development of Germ Theory and the Rise of Modern Vaccinology

Jenner's discovery, while groundbreaking, was based on empirical observation rather than a scientific understanding of disease.

It wasn't until the development of germ theory in the mid-19th century that the science of vaccinology began to take shape.

Germ theory, championed by scientists such as Louis Pasteur and Robert Koch, proposed that microorganisms were the cause of many diseases. This theory laid the groundwork for understanding how vaccines work—by stimulating the immune system to recognize and combat these disease-causing microbes.

Louis Pasteur, a French microbiologist and chemist, made significant contributions to vaccine development. In the 1880s, Pasteur developed vaccines for two major diseases: chicken cholera and anthrax. His method, called "attenuation", involved weakening the virulent form of a pathogen so that it could no longer cause disease but would still stimulate an immune response.

Pasteur's most famous work in vaccination was his development of a rabies vaccine in 1885. Rabies was a deadly disease, and there was no known treatment. Pasteur used a weakened form of the virus to inoculate Joseph Meister, a young boy who had been bitten by a rabid dog. The vaccine was successful, and the boy survived, marking the first successful use of a vaccine to treat an infection after exposure to the disease.

Early 20th Century: Expansion of Vaccine Science

The early 20th century saw a rapid expansion in vaccine development. This period was characterized by the development of vaccines for several infectious diseases, many of which had been major causes of morbidity and mortality.

One of the earliest vaccines developed in the 20th century was the vaccine for diphtheria. The diphtheria toxoid vaccine was introduced in 1923, and worked by using a chemically inactivated form of the toxin produced by the diphtheria bacterium. This method allowed the immune system to build immunity without causing disease. The success of this vaccine was monumental in reducing the incidence of diphtheria, particularly in children.

In 1926, a vaccine for whooping cough (pertussis) was developed, and it was later combined with the diphtheria and tetanus vaccines to form the DTP vaccine in the 1940s. The combination vaccine made it easier to immunize large populations against multiple diseases.

Another significant milestone in the early 20th century was the development of the tuberculosis (TB) vaccine. In 1921, Albert Calmette and Camille Guérin developed the Bacillus Calmette-Guérin (BCG) vaccine, which remains one of the most widely used vaccines in the world, particularly in countries with high rates of tuberculosis.

The Era of Viral Vaccines: Polio, Measles, and Mumps

The mid-20th century marked the dawn of viral vaccines, which were developed using inactivated or weakened forms of viruses. One of the most notable achievements during this time was the development of the polio vaccine.

Polio was a devastating disease, particularly in the first half of the 20th century, causing paralysis and death, especially among children. In 1955, Jonas Salk introduced the first inactivated polio vaccine (IPV), which used a killed version of the virus to stimulate immunity. A few years later, Albert Sabin developed an oral polio vaccine (OPV) using a live, attenuated form of the virus. The introduction of these vaccines led to the near-global eradication of polio.

During the same period, vaccines for other viral diseases were developed. In 1963, John Enders and Thomas Peebles developed the measles vaccine, which was followed by vaccines for mumps in 1967 and rubella in 1969. These vaccines were later combined into the MMR vaccine (measles, mumps, and rubella), which became a cornerstone of childhood immunization programs around the world.

The success of the polio and MMR vaccines marked a new era in public health, as widespread vaccination campaigns led to a dramatic decline in the incidence of these diseases. Vaccine development continued to advance, with new vaccines being introduced for diseases like hepatitis B (1981) and chickenpox (1995).

The Vaccine Controversies and Challenges

Despite their overwhelming success, vaccines have not been without controversy. One of the earliest instances of vaccine opposition occurred in the 19th century with the introduction of the smallpox vaccination. Some people objected to vaccination on religious or philosophical grounds, while others were concerned about the safety and effectiveness of the procedure.

In the late 20th century, vaccine safety concerns resurfaced with the publication of a now-discredited study by Andrew Wakefield in 1998, which falsely claimed a link between the MMR vaccine and autism. Despite extensive scientific evidence disproving this claim, the study fueled vaccine hesitancy and led to a decline in vaccination rates in some countries, resulting in outbreaks of measles and other vaccine-preventable diseases.

Addressing vaccine hesitancy and ensuring public trust in vaccination programs remains a challenge in modern medicine. Efforts to combat misinformation, improve vaccine access, and promote education about the benefits of vaccination are essential to maintaining high vaccination coverage and preventing the resurgence of infectious diseases.

The 21st Century and the COVID-19 Pandemic: A New Era in Vaccinology

The 21st century has brought significant advancements in vaccine technology. One of the most notable developments is the use of genetic and molecular techniques to create new types of vaccines, such as DNA, RNA, and viral vector vaccines.

The COVID-19 pandemic, which began in late 2019, accelerated the development and deployment of these new vaccine technologies. The Pfizer-BioNTech and Moderna COVID-19 vaccines, both based on messenger RNA (mRNA) technology, were the first mRNA vaccines approved for use in humans. These vaccines work by delivering genetic instructions to cells, prompting them to produce a protein found on the surface of the virus. This protein triggers an immune response without causing disease.

The speed at which these vaccines were developed and distributed was unprecedented. The global scientific community mobilized to create, test, and approve COVID-19 vaccines in record time, leading to the widespread immunization of millions of people worldwide. The success of mRNA vaccines has opened the door to new possibilities for vaccine development, including vaccines for other viral infections, cancer, and autoimmune diseases.

The Future of Vaccines

As we move further into the 21st century, vaccine development continues to evolve. Advances in biotechnology, genomics, and synthetic biology are enabling the creation of more precise and effective vaccines. Scientists are exploring new delivery methods, such as needle-free vaccines and oral vaccines, which could improve access and acceptance, particularly in low-resource settings.

Additionally, research into universal vaccines—such as a universal influenza vaccine that could protect against all strains of the flu—is ongoing. These vaccines hold the potential to provide long-lasting protection and eliminate the need for annual immunization campaigns.

The history of vaccine development is a testament to human ingenuity and the power of science. From the early days of variolation to the development of mRNA vaccines, vaccines have played an indispensable role in protecting public health and shaping the course of human history. As new challenges emerge, the ongoing research and innovation in vaccine science will continue to be vital in addressing both existing and emerging infectious diseases. With the rapid advancements in technology and a deeper understanding of immunology, the future of vaccinology holds great promise. Whether combating long-standing diseases or preparing for future pandemics, vaccines will remain a cornerstone of global health, helping to safeguard populations and improve the quality of life for people around the world. Through continued research, international collaboration, and public health initiatives, we can hope to overcome many of the challenges that still face vaccine development, ensuring that future generations are protected from preventable diseases.

6

WHAT IS IN THESE SHOTS ANYWAY?

THIS IS THE PART OF THE story that goes above and beyond my expertise. For the record, I do not have a background in molecular biology, and although I do have a background in toxicology, I am not a molecular biologist or toxicologist—so it's a good thing I know one of the best! Her name is Dr. Janci Lindsay. Her biography highlights just how qualified she is. It states, "Dr. Janci Chunn Lindsay is the Director of Toxicology and Molecular Biology for Toxicology Support Services, LLC. She holds a doctorate (PhD) in Biochemistry and Molecular Biology from the University of Texas Graduate School of Biomedical Sciences, M.D. Anderson Cancer Center, Houston.

"Dr. Lindsay has extensive experience in analyzing the molecular profile of pharmacologic responses as they pertain to the dose/response relationship. Her expertise centers on evaluating the complex dynamics of toxicity, such as toxicant pharmacology, exposure route, host metabolism, and subsequent cellular effects as they relate to the contribution of specific substances to impairment, health risk, or human disease."

What does all that mean? It means she's super smart when it comes to microbiology, and she offers some of the best insight into the unknown when it comes to Covid shots. She's also very plugged in as many other experts have consulted her since the pandemic began, and her Rolodex is very extensive. She has over 30 years of experience in the industry and became a fixture on the Covid map when she started to speak out about what she was seeing in practice regarding these new "vaccines". I had the pleasure of interviewing her at length, and she has become a friend.

We discussed how most people look at a vial of this clear liquid and think of all the other "vaccines" they've gotten over the years. If it's being touted by the government as "safe and effective" and everybody's doing it, why not get one for yourself. However, if you knew what was inside that clear liquid, you may think twice about putting it into your arm. If you look up what's in these shots as reported by one of the manufacturers, the information can be a tad bit confusing. The following is what Pfizer reports is inside their shots:

"Pfizer-BioNTech COVID-19 Vaccine contains the following ingredients: messenger ribonucleic acid (mRNA), lipids (((4-hydroxybutyl) azanediyl) bis (hexane-6,1-diyl) bis (2- hexyldecanoate), 2 [(polyethylene glycol)-2000]-N,N-ditetradecylacetamide, 1,2-distearoyl-sn-glycero-3-phosphocholine, and cholesterol), tromethamine, tromethamine hydrochloride, and sucrose. Pfizer-BioNTech COVID-19 Vaccine may also contain sodium chloride."

I think if most people look at that list of ingredients, their brain may just shut off completely. It looks like a list of ingredients you may find on the back of a lawn fertilizer bag. In other words, you'd most likely need a degree in molecular biology to decipher all that! It's hard enough trying to figure out what's in these things before delving into what they are doing to the human body in practice. The answer appears to be two-fold and conflated because the answer to the latter question helps us understand better what is in these things, and of course, the bigger question is why?

To break down these ingredients into lay terms, the definitions of these categories would look like this:

mRNA vaccines (Pfizer-BioNTech and Moderna)

Messenger ribonucleic acid (mRNA): This is the key ingredient that teaches your cells how to make a protein that triggers an immune response to the virus.

- **Lipids (fats):** These help to protect the mRNA and deliver it into your cells.
- **Salts (such as sodium chloride) and sugars (such as sucrose):** These help to maintain the stability of the vaccine.
- **Acids (such as acetic acid) and acid stabilizers (such as tromethamine):** These help to keep the vaccine at the right acidity level.

I asked Dr. Lindsay where one even starts in all of this, since this topic can be overwhelming and confusing. She had just gotten off a phone call with a group of scientists and an IRB to speak about getting gamete studies started. What are gamete studies? They test to see if the DNA of these Covid shots was being integrated or passed onto the sperm or ova. This is extremely important because Kevin McKernan and a group over in Europe discovered that sequences were integrated from the plasmids that have contaminated the mRNA vaccines at chromosomes 9 and 12. Granted, this is a cancer cell line, but it's extremely important to see if this is happening in our next generation in gametes. For those of you without a background in biology, a gamete is a reproductive cell of an animal or plant. In animals, female gametes are called ova or egg cells. Male gametes are called sperm.

"Wait," I said, "so these shots that people are receiving can somehow change their DNA?" Dr. Lindsay responded, "Yes, they can." For a long time, it has been known that gene therapy carries the inherent risk of something called insertional mutagenesis. DNA that's being used in gene therapy can be incorporated into your own genome. Most of the time when this happens, it doesn't happen functionally. In other words, you don't get the gene, however, in gene therapy, it's a little more targeted to become integrated. Often it becomes broken so that just little pieces will be integrated, or it will become integrated non-functionally, or it may sit above an oncogene or inhibit a tumor suppressor. The problem with all this is that insertional mutagenesis can lead to cancer! So, if you have cancer or a rare disease that is incurable, the risk versus reward would suggest trying this therapy, but otherwise, no perfectly healthy individual would ever be selected for this type of treatment. Here's the kicker, in the old days, the people performing this type of treatment would make the individual receiving the treatment become sterilized before receiving it so that the recipient would not inadvertently transfer this to the next generation... Yes, they sterilized anyone getting this treatment to protect future generations of humans.

This brings us to our next topic, what is an Oncovirus and what in the world is SV40? An oncovirus or oncogenic virus is a virus that can cause cancer. This is a DNA or RNA genome causing cancer, and can sometimes be referred to as a "tumor virus" or "cancer virus". SV40 happens to be one such oncovirus; however, much debate has been made over whether or not it's been a culprit for cancer over the course of many decades. SV40 virus or Simian Virus 40 is a polyomavirus that sometimes causes tumors. It is found in both monkeys and humans. It can cause tumors in animals but most often persists as a latent infection. Between 1955 and 1961, it was discovered that there was contamination in polio vaccine batches with the SV40 virus. This led to suspicion that an increase of cancer would occur and that these polio vaccines were to blame.

The SV40 virus is not an oncovirus to the African Green Monkey, it's host. The monkeys have gotten used to this virus and they have mounted defenses accordingly. However, scientists were using the kidney cells of these monkeys to grow the polio vaccines back in the 1950s. This is where the story may have started, as scientists discovered that these monkeys carried many different diseases, and SV40 was just one of them. SV40 happens to cause cancer in other animals as well, like hamsters, in addition to humans. This was all discovered after the Qatar incident, where the polio vaccines were not attenuated correctly and gave the recipients polio. When this happened, the vaccine was studied more in depth, which revealed the presence of SV40. As I've mentioned in previous works, not all "vaccines" are the same. When attenuated correctly and administered without contaminants, the polio vaccines have been attributed to saving more than 20 million people from paralysis and 1.5 million childhood deaths. The larger issue is that the major differences in vaccination technology are not explained, and it's too often that someone wants to argue the effectiveness of "vaccines" with me by pointing out polio... They are NOT the same type of inoculations!

While only 10 to 30% of the polio vaccines were known to have been contaminated with SV40, governments were hesitant to tell people of this little snafu as they thought it would cause worldwide vaccine hesitancy. However, the fact that they infected millions of people with the SV40 virus was the cause for an alarming rise in cancer over the next few decades. So, I asked Dr. Lindsay, "Are you saying we have found sequences of

SV40 in these Covid shots?" Her response gets into the weeds a bit with the science, but the conclusion is terrifying. Dr. Lindsay responded, "So this is really interesting. They purported that they only used the plasmids and the mRNA vaccines to make lots and lots of copies of the DNA. They wanted to scale up and make enough of this DNA that they would reverse transcribe to the mRNA. In the reverse transcription step, they would add the synthetic uracil and incorporate that. But to make enough of this DNA, instead of doing it on the synthesizers, which is really expensive and time-consuming, they would just make billions of copies in E. Coli by using plasmids."

"DNA plasmids are essentially like little copy machines," Dr Lindsay continued, "However, if they just wanted to do that, they would have put the bacterial sequences that allowed for replication in bacteria." These companies were trying to make these copies as quickly as possible to keep up with the demand of the public and the government citing Covid as a global health risk. I'm sure you recall the narrative at the time that this was a "pandemic of the unvaccinated." These companies should have been using a bacterial promoter but instead opted for an SV40 promoter, an SV40 nuclear targeting sequence. There was simply no need to do that because bacteria cannot use an SV40 promoter. Dr Lindsay continued, "So they were trying to target the human nucleus, why would you add a nuclear targeting sequence to this if you were not?" This is where the story gets scary. It points to something nefarious and planned because somebody would have had to make the decision to do exactly that.

It's not just a "somebody" in this instance, but it seems to be a coordinated effort across all the pharmaceutical companies. This is the point in the story where my knowledge of testing and treatment finally combined with that of another expert, and a brighter lightbulb went off in the room. I have written about virology and how viruses transmit, the effectiveness of the "vaccines" versus natural immunity, and the who, what, where, when, and why. I explained about what is inside the capsicum of a virus in my previous book. There are about 27 cells inside the envelope of this virus, and when you get Covid, you would naturally develop B and T lymphocytes to the entirety of the virus. This means that the next time you catch Covid, when the spike protein mutates enough to fool the body, you will have memory cells for most of the proteins in the virus. Essentially, you are now getting a reaction to the new spike protein, and the symptomatology can vary widely between different spikes.

If you had asked me to develop an inoculation in a vacuum, my limited knowledge would tell me to target the whole of the virus, not the spike protein. The spike protein changes so much and so often that if I were to target the spike, all I would be doing was essentially creating a "flu shot." We've been telling our patients exactly that—these "vaccines" work like flu shots—and we have recorded an average antibody response of around 120 days. In other words, like flu shots, they give you antibodies to the spike but not the entirety of the virus. This research is based on our own 19,000 patients and why we did NOT recommend these shots for Covid. The main two reasons were, again, we didn't lose any patients during the pandemic, and the shots didn't work. So why in good faith would we "recommend" something experimental that our patients didn't need and with a shot that didn't work?

I asked Dr. Lindsay, "Do you think this was done on purpose?" She responded, "Yes, this was done on purpose to promote integration of the sequence in the plasmid." She continued with emphasis, "They hid things from the regulators, they omitted SV40 sequences from the plasmid maps." Plasmid maps had to be submitted to the regulators, and all these companies, in unison, left out vital information from the plasmid maps. They failed to include them in the EMA, the TGA, and the FDA presentations. That points to a coordinated effort, and one with nefarious intent.

Dr. Lindsay explained why there was so much hesitation in rolling out this type of technology before the pandemic appeared. "So, the reason this technology never came to market, even though it was over 40 years old, was because of the risks of Leukemia, lymphomas, and lethal autoimmune diseases, and trying to get your cells to express this particular protein, they would have lethal autoimmune reactions." We have seen in practice with our patient population that these shots cause an abundance of issues, including heart, joint, and autoimmune disorders. They cause an inflammatory reaction to a patient in an area of susceptibility and can cause an exacerbation of an issue that may not have been present before administration. Dr. Lindsay explains it like this, "They suppress your immune system. We know that when your immune system is depressed, it is unable to keep cancer in check. We all have cancer all the time. We all have lots of cancer clones hanging around. It's our immune system that keeps those cancers in check and keeps us from developing cancer. This is why when you have immune deficiencies like AIDS, or anything that impacts your immune system severely, the result is that you will develop cancer."

What's more alarming is that scientists knew about the harms that these spike proteins caused even before the vaccines rolled out. In the fall of 2019, scientists found that if you injected recombinant spike protein into humanized mice, they got spontaneous thrombosis. What does that all mean? A humanized mouse is a genetically modified mouse that has functioning human genes and cells. A lot of our knowledge about several human biological processes has been obtained from studying animal models like rodents and non-human primates. The mouse immune systems are humanized by irradiating and destroying the host immune system and introducing human immune cells. Humanized mouse models are used to compare tumor therapies, study the human immune system, and to study the function of genes in healthy and diseased models.

When it came to these humanized mice, the researchers tried to isolate what was harming people who got COVID-19. They found that if they took the spike protein from the virus, and they made it recombinantly, then injected it into these mice, it gave them disseminated blood clotting! As Dr. Lindsay remarked, "Doesn't that sound like a great thing to inject into billions of people just a few months later?" We know that Covid causes clotting, and we know that these "vaccines" cause clotting, and as I've mentioned in previous writings, we weren't checking people's clotting factors by doing D-Dimer testing before injecting them with these shots. Medicine has never been one-size-fits-all, yet this is the approach the entirety of the medical community was taking during the pandemic—again, for a shot that doesn't work and for a virus that was and is 99.98 survivable without any treatment. Does that sound like a reasonable approach to you?

So, what else is inside that clear liquid that's getting injected into your arm? It gets a little scientific, but I'll try to break it down for you. We can start with the lipid nanoparticle, which is four different lipids combined in a fat bubble, essentially to help it get into and past cell membranes. Lipids are fatty compounds that perform a variety of functions in your body. Lipid nanoparticles are a novel pharmaceutical drug delivery system that were first approved in 2018 but became more well-known during the COVID-19 pandemic. The fact that these lipids were designed to pass nuclear membranes was another thing that wasn't disclosed to regulators.

As I mentioned earlier, the big question is, why didn't some of the companies manufacturing these "vaccines" use the nucleocapsid of the virus? The spike sequence of the virus is changing and mutating all the time, so why would you choose that as your region? It's far more susceptible to mutation than the nucleocapsid, or the whole of the virus. Wouldn't you choose something that didn't necessitate changing and making shots all the time? If you were going to develop a true vaccine, then absolutely you would!

This was my issue when these "vaccines" first rolled out. We weren't recommending them because we knew this, but we also discovered how short the lifespan was. When we called patients to notify them of a positive status, they would often gasp in non-belief because they had been "fully vaccinated". We warned our patients that they would need multiple shots and need them year after year, sometimes multiple shots per year for there to be any resistant effect to Covid. But that's not what the government and media were touting on national television. If you recall, the initial effectiveness estimates were between 77% and 95% between J&J and Moderna and Pfizer respectively. I asked Dr. Lindsay about natural immunity and if it is indeed stronger than what the shots provide, and she responded, "Yeah, so with your natural immunity, you're right. You get the B cell immunity, mucosal immunity, and humoral immunity as well. Whereas you inject these, so you're bypassing your mucosal immunity, and you're also using something that is mutating, it's not even relevant after a few months. You are also forcing the further mutation of the virus when you get it."

If we knew this and experts like Dr. Lindsay knew this, it leads me to believe that others in the administration, the FDA, and the CDC knew all this as well. This leads me back to zeroing in on nefarious behavior. Why would the FDA try to hide clinical data from you for 75 years if everything was above board? Why would the Department of Justice be stepping in on behalf of the FDA? Why would there be amendments made to the FD&C (Federal Food, Drug and Cosmetic Act) code that allowed for adulteration and misbranding specifically, and no CGMP (Current Good Manufacturing Practices) of these shots?

Dr. Lindsay added, "These are DOD countermeasures. That's how they're classified. You can go to the FDA page and see they're under emergency use authorization under 21 CFR, Code of Federal Regulations, 360 BBB, through 3A. That is the medical countermeasures amendment that has been added to the FD&C code. Why would they stipulate adulterated and misbranded? I mean, essentially, you're saying that you could add arsenic to them if you wanted." The code says that these shots will not be unapproved, and furthermore, they will be licensed by the FDA. These are measures that allow them to rush things through, adulterate, or do anything they really want with the final product, and in turn, hide the data for 75 years!

I know that the word nefarious can have you thinking that I or those contributing to this work have gone down a rabbit hole, but there are two ways of thinking of this. They are either nefarious in nature, and they want to hide the data, or they hurried it through so quickly that they don't want to be liable for anything that arises, since we were forcing this on the whole of the population. However, remember that this is a coronavirus with a mortality rate that is less than that of influenza. We used an experimental gene technology, in which we learned quickly about the myocarditis and clotting issues patients were having—and no-one investigated? The people pulling the strings were and still are, at the time of this writing, touting new and improved boosters. This looks like it was weaponized, especially with the cognitive distortion associated with ignoring clear and present data. Dr. Lindsay adds, "I'll be extremely clear that this is a bioweapon that is meant to depopulate, but they are trying to make a little bit of money along the way. So, it's not meant to kill you right away, but give you cancer, give you prion disease, give you a cardiac disease, myocarditis, a variety of diseases, and blood clots along the way so they can make a buck."

Dr. Lindsay and I were talking about the increase in the amount of cancer centers opening all over the world. This was reminiscent of a conversation I had recently had with Edward Dowd. I had just had Edward as a guest on my show about a week before my conversation with Dr. Lindsay, and he was saying exactly the same thing. Traditionally, there really wasn't much money in cancer, as morbid as that may sound, but when you go to school all those years to practice medicine, you've got to find a way to pay those student loans back. Cancer has never been much of a cash cow in medicine, but Dr. Lindsay and Edward Dowd are correct, the amount of new cancer centers is astounding. Is there a link to what is happening now to these shots that rolled out worldwide? We'll get more in depth into that once you hear what the practitioners are starting to see at ground level.

So what if you never got one of these shots but your parents did, could that mean a child born to a "vaccinated person" would in turn have spike protein running around in their system? The short answer is yes. There's a couple of different ways that could happen. The first is called sperm-mediated gene transfer. This is an interesting phenomenon, and it's the same way scientists made a kind of dirty transgenic variation of a mouse a long time ago. They would incubate some DNA with some mouse sperm. The sperm would pick it up, but they wouldn't generate the DNA, it would be tethered extra chromosomally, kind of like its own plasmid. The sperm would fertilize the egg, and it would still be tethered extra chromosomally, so you would end up with mosaic offspring. This genetic expression would decrease later in life, but it could continue for one generation. However, some of the cells would then be making the spike protein that would have their own plasmids. These were essentially circular DNA pieces that were just making the plasmid or making the spike protein repeatedly. So, the short answer to the question of whether this could pass from generation to generation is yes, but for females, this is even worse. Females are born with all the eggs they'll ever have; they don't produce new ones as life continues. If the expression propagated to the female, she would inherently pass it onto her offspring. For men, we would hope that this is transient.

Dr. Lindsay and I continued our conversation. I told her that while we were doing thousands of tests at assisted livings and police departments weekly, one of our clients had asked us to conduct occasional antibody tests on a group that had been vaccinated. We obliged, and I was thankful for the wealth of knowledge the data would give our company. This was one aspect of Covid that we weren't studying, and the data would allow us to compare antibody data from the shot to that of natural immunity. The average came out to be about 120 days or 4 months of active antibodies in the blood after "vaccination". This told us a few things. One, that these shots didn't really work, or they were working like a flu shot. We also found that some patients had high levels for as long as a year, and some only for a few weeks. This could have been dependent on which type of "vaccine" they were receiving, how it was stored and handled, etc., but we didn't have access to all that information. This was a broad look at what a patient had in their blood over the course of time.

Dr. Lindsay asked a very pertinent question, she said, "For how many different vaccines do you measure your steady state antibody levels?" I paused for a second and thought about it before Dr. Lindsay jumped back in, "And if you don't have those antibody levels circulating around for everything that you've been vaccinated to, do you not have immunity? You're not going to have significant levels of antibodies until you have a serious infection, it's just another way to get people to get more vaccines! Can you imagine having antibodies to everything you've ever been immunized to circulating through our blood all the time at significant levels? They would get tangled up and you'd have constant autoimmune reactions"

There is so much to delve into when it comes to the different types of "vaccines", all the lot numbers, and what the potential dangers are from putting these into your system. There is even a site online where you can reference specific lot numbers of these shots to see how many VAERS cases were reported and for what. Howbadismybatch.com is one of these sites. If you have your lot numbers from the shots you were given, it gives you a little insight into how bad that specific batch may have been. Of course, if you recall the chapter on how VAERS works, keep in mind that this information is just a snapshot of what is potentially out there.

Just this week, at the time of writing, a new study came out of Japan showing an uptick in cancer diagnoses nationwide after the vaccine rollout. Another study showed that people with three or more vaccinations were more susceptible to getting Covid. When you understand symptomatology and testing, this makes perfect sense, as those with multiple inflammatory reactions to shots can become more susceptible to cytokine storm, and those getting sick may be more likely to receive a Covid test or respiratory pathogen panel.

It will take years before the full picture of the data is presented and understood, and that's if the mainstream media will even report on it. It will be years before the public has any idea of the harm these shots, that were so hastily rushed to market, have caused the whole of humanity. But if you listen to the heroes who stick their necks out to try and warn you, like Dr. Janci Lindsay, you'll be well ahead of the curve.

7

SUDDEN DEATHS

YOU MAY HAVE SEEN OR HEARD of the documentary *Died Suddenly*. It's a film about an embalmer who started seeing anomalies while trying to embalm the deceased, finding resistance when forcing the embalming fluid into the arteries of bodies. Upon further investigation, he discovered white fibrous substances that took the shape of and were blocking the arteries.

He claims these clots are different from what he had typically encountered previously in his career, and associates their occurrence with the period following the introduction of COVID-19 vaccines. His observations and conclusions have been embraced by certain anti-vaccine communities, but they have also sparked significant controversy and criticism from medical experts. That last sentence should spark your interest, since most of the "medical experts" had gotten Covid completely wrong. It was the people yelling "smoke" who eventually led us to the fire, and Richard Hirschman's claims should not fall on deaf ears—otherwise, this fire may burn uncontrollably.

Hirschman's claims have not been supported by peer-reviewed scientific evidence, and several experts have expressed skepticism regarding the connection between the clots and COVID-19 vaccines. However, I have had my own share of naysayers who don't do what I do for a living, and those detractors didn't collect a fraction of the data I derived during the pandemic. I wanted to hear it from the horse's mouth, so to speak, and see if we could make heads or tails of the reports before arriving at any conclusions. Nonetheless, critics, including medical professionals and fact-checking organizations, argue that the formation of clots can vary depending on numerous factors, such as the location in the body and time elapsed since death, making it difficult to definitively link these clots to vaccines. Additionally, the lab analysis of these clots has been questioned for its lack of rigor and transparency. Despite this, Hirschman continues to advocate for further investigation into the phenomenon, citing concerns for public health.

So what is an embalmer, and what exactly do they do? Embalmers are professionals trained in the preservation and preparation of deceased bodies for funerals and other ceremonies. Their primary task is to prevent decomposition and ensure that the body is presented in a dignified and natural state for viewing. This is typically achieved through a process called embalming, where the blood is removed from the body and replaced with preservative fluids, usually formaldehyde-based solutions, that delay the breakdown of tissues. Embalmers also clean and disinfect the body, set facial features to create a peaceful appearance, and can restore and reconstruct damaged areas of the body, especially in cases of trauma, to ensure the deceased looks as natural as possible.

In addition to technical work, embalmers play a significant emotional role in helping families cope with loss. They often work closely with funeral directors to prepare the body according to the wishes of the family or religious customs. Embalmers may also offer cosmetic services such as applying makeup, hairstyling, and dressing the deceased in their chosen attire. Their expertise ensures that the body is preserved long enough for the funeral or memorial services to take place, allowing families the opportunity to say their final goodbyes.

I had the opportunity to interview Richard Hirschman personally to try and get to the bottom of this strange phenomenon, and what I found was astounding! First off, Richard has been in the profession of embalming or funeral directing for the better part of 20 years. His reputation is impeccable, and his dedication to his craft and to the families of the loved ones being serviced shines through when speaking to him or the people who know him best. I had reached out to a few funeral directors for guidance on this topic and was met with silence. Richard told me why that may be. He said, "In the funeral business, we are trained early on that what happens in the funeral home, especially the embalming room, stays in the embalming room." Funeral directors and embalmers deal with sensitive family information, considering the circumstances, and no family would want stories of their loved one coming out publicly. Richard was very careful early on when talking about this phenomenon to other people, making sure that no one could identify the deceased and risk some ethical breach. Richard explained, "It's a firable offense if you talk about things that are happening in the embalming room publicly, so there is a fear of somebody getting fired for speaking out." With a 20-year career on the line, Richard was trepidatious at best to speak out publicly about what he was seeing. Richard stated that he knows another embalmer who had spoken out and had her license suspended. He also mentions another who was told that if she wanted to keep her license, she would cease and desist with any talk outside the embalming room. Let's not forget that the government controls the licensure, and well, need I say more?

One thing I can say about Richard is he is a straight shooter. He tells it like it is and doesn't hold a lot back. His passion for his work and desire to want to correct the record about what's been reported on this subject is abundant. He didn't strike me as somebody who was interested in publicity or had a desire to be in front of a camera. Richard truly cares about his craft and the families he works for; it shines through when you get to know him. The detractors may want to discount these reports, but for Richard, this was a leap, far away from the norm of everyday life, it was the act of a whistleblower, if you will. However, the government doesn't often protect whistleblowers when they go against the grain of the entire narrative. Richard stated, "We're witnessing Nazi Germany all over again in a sense. We're finding out who would truly speak up to help those in need and who would remain silent to allow people to be led to their concentration camp."

Richard mentions Major Tom Haviland, a retired United States Air Force officer who conducted an anonymous survey where 66 percent of embalmers reported seeing these white fibrous clots. He did a follow-up survey, where an astounding 73 percent reported seeing them. It seems that while the mainstream media and "safe and effective" narrative proponents want to discredit Richard Hirschman, realistically, his reports may be just the tip of the iceberg. Why are these reports ignored by the mainstream media? If you talk to the public about these phenomena, most will admit to having never heard about them. It's the curious individuals who seek out alternative media that have any sense of what is really happening, and that these, in fact, are related to the mass vaccinations conducted after the COVID-19 outbreak. All these discoveries started in 2021 and coincided with the "vaccine" rollouts.

2020 Clots Look a Lot Different...

The onset of COVID-19 started causing people to clot, and as I've said before, both natural COVID-19 and the COVID-19 "vaccines" cause clots. But, as Richard told us, in the embalming room, they are very different. Richard stated, "We did see an increase in clotting in 2020, but it wasn't these white fibrous things." To put things into context, all of Richard Hirschman's work is conducted in Alabama, but he does belong to associations and often speaks with colleagues around the country. What Richard was seeing in 2020 on the embalming table were gritty little clots or typical blood clots that look like sand when they come out onto the table. This story remains consistent with his colleagues around the country and from multiple reports around the world.

Richard then pulled out a jar with a very large, white, string like clot in it. He said, "This particular one came out of an artery. It's 18 inches long." Richard said they never used to get clots out of arteries, they used to see them only in veins, but the blood clots were typically red and kind of gritty. They usually broke right up as they came out on the embalming table. These new kinds of clots are completely different. They don't look like they are made up of red blood cells, and if they are not, what in the world could they be made of? Richard sent me a scientific analysis conducted of the materials coming out of the deceased. While there are over 500 proteins found, I will list the top 21 with their rank and respective percentage of material:

1	Fibrinogen beta chain	35.2848 %
2	Fibrinogen gamma chain	16.0694 %
3	Hemoglobin subunit beta	14.0401 %
4	Fibrinogen alpha chain	4.5841 %
5	Hemoglobin subunit alpha	2.8530 %
6	Actin, cytoplasmic 1	2.6850 %
7	Immunoglobulin heavy constant gamma 1	2.0120 %
8	Fibronectin	1.1841 %

9	Myeloperoxidase	1.1448 %
10	Cathepsin G	0.9065 %
11	Integrin alpha IIb	0.8033 %
12	Coagulation factor XIII A chain	0.6776 %
13	Vitronectin	0.6020 %
14	Band 3 anion transport protein	0.5974 %
15	Alpha-2-macroglobuin	0.5874 %
16	Glyceraldehyde-3-phosphate dehydrogenase	0.4735 %
17	Immunoglobulin heavy constant gamma 2	0.3920 %
18	Neutrophil elastase	0.3626 %
19	Filamin-A	0.3431 %
20	Complement C3	0.3384 %
21	von Willebrand factor	0.2784 %

I've said it many times, but "when you're explaining, you're losing." Having to explain this chemistry to the public is a daunting task. People only seem to care about those calamari-like substances if they are being removed from a loved one's body. We now have a scientific analysis of the substances; the next logical question is, what in the world is causing them?

We had a clue as early as June 2021, but you probably never heard about it through the mainstream media. The American College of Cardiology published a paper referencing "Vaccine-induced Thrombotic Thrombocytopenia (VITT) and COVID-19 Vaccines: What Cardiovascular Clinicians Need to Know." Another paper published by The *New England Journal of Medicine* in August 2021 was titled "Clinical Features of Vaccine-Induced Immune Thrombocytopenia and Thrombosis." The latter states, "VITT is rare, with an incidence of 14.9 per million after the first or unknown dose of COVID-19 vaccine, and 1.8 cases per million after second doses." The article later says, "VITT can affect people of all ages, but summary data from UK yellow card reporting indicate that after a first dose, the incidence rate in adults aged 18–49 years is twice that of adults 50 years and older." In other words, younger people had higher incidence rates of clotting from a shot they never needed in the first place. The article continues, "The guideline emphasizes the importance of providing information to vaccine recipients to help them recognize common and unusual symptoms arising from COVID-19 vaccination and to know when and how to seek help." Another article in PubMed Central, July 2021, titled "Vaccine-induced immune thrombotic thrombocytopenia (VITT), reaction to COVID-19 vaccines", states a "high risk of death from venous or arterial thrombosis or secondary hemorrhage." All this evidence came out relatively early, but somehow the public "missed" it. The media kept citing the government's narrative that these shots were "safe and effective".

The data I derived from testing and treating over 19,000 patients was enough to paint a graphic picture of the effectiveness of those shots, but somehow that information was censored as well. When you talk to patients every day about their symptoms, track their recovery time, and put real values on the metrics being collected, it was easy to conclude that the "vaccines" weren't effective at all. This again was the reason we never recommended them to our patients. The "safe" part of the equation needed a little more time to be studied, but if we actually "followed the science", we would have seen that the indicators were already out there and what Richard discovered on the embalming table already had a very reasonable explanation. In fact, yet another peer reviewed study from October 13, 2021, states, "SARS-CoV-2 spike protein induces abnormal inflammatory blood clots neutralized by fibrin immunotherapy." A one sentence summary of the article reads, "SARS-CoV-2 spike induces structurally abnormal blood clots and thrombo-inflammation neutralized by a fibrin-targeted antibody."

Richard Hirschman had been proven right long before he started blowing the whistle on the anomalies he was seeing and still sees. The proof was already being studied and published that SARS-CoV-2 spike with fibrinogen and fibrin resulted in abnormal blood clot formations. The spike protein is a fibrinogen binding partner and provides a mechanism basis for the formation of abnormal clots—or the stringy, calamari-like substances that Richard felt he needed to alert the public about.

Richard states that in 2020, his industry started seeing an increase in "normal" clotting but in an abundance of patients coming in from the hospitals. Richard doesn't know exactly why that is but stated, "Looking back on it now, it was probably from some of the medications that the patients were being put on, most likely because their kidneys were shut down from the use of Remdesivir and treatments like that." He continued, "Some of them had so much edema, you almost couldn't identify the individual. They looked nothing like themselves, and there wasn't much we could do. So, there was an increase in clotting, but it was still typically just more of the traditional red, jelly-like clots. Then January 2021 came along, and that's when all hell broke loose."

Richard's funeral home got so busy so fast and, of course, the narrative was to attribute it all to Covid, further adding to the fear of the nation. Richard said that the pileup eventually started to slow down in February and March, but in April 2021, the strange stuff started to occur. April 2021 was when he started to notice these new kinds of clots. Richard stated, "It was every once in a while, it wasn't all the time. The first time I remember was on an axillary or brachial. I had to use the axillary because the arm wasn't getting fluid, so I went ahead and cut into it. When I cut the artery, I could see something in there and I pulled it out." He said he just found it really strange, but as time went on, he kept seeing them, and they not only became more abundant, but they became more robust as well. As this continued throughout the summer of 2021, he started asking his colleagues if they were encountering the same things. Richard stated, "Some of these people had 30, 40 and even 50 years of experience. I would bring them over to the embalming table and show them these strange clots. I was trying to make sure I wasn't crazy."

He continued, "In September 2021, I had a man in his early 50s, he had a massive, white fibrous clot that was almost the length of his leg. I didn't measure it, but I was asked to take a picture of it because the funeral director thought it was the craziest thing he'd ever seen and wanted to send it to his brother, who is also an embalmer. That started my documentation of what I was seeing." Richard was so perplexed that he began looking up images of different thrombosis and blood clots just to see if he could finally identify what he was witnessing, now on a mass scale, but to no avail. The closest thing he could find was a substance that develops around a PICC line, where it comes out coated with a white substance, but there was no real correlation.

Richard showed me a clot that came out of a leg that was 48 inches long. Imagine something like that developing in your body due to an inflammatory reaction we now know exists. The question I had was whether these develop postmortem, or can they start developing in the body while the blood is still flowing and be the actual cause of death? Richard tells me that there are other whistleblowers who have pulled out these substances during surgery. One doctor stated that in all the cases he had seen as a vascular surgeon, 99 percent of them were in people who had received the COVID-19 shots. Richard didn't have to convince me any further that this is indeed happening in the living. My initial hypothesis was that these could not develop the structure they had attained within hours of the patient passing. Tom Haviland's name came up again. Remember the Major from the Air Force who did an anonymous survey of funeral homes? Tom decided he would like to conduct a survey of vascular surgeons to start gathering information, but he was met with resistance. Apparently, he was told by a large group that there would be no participation, which really raises an eyebrow.

Where I come from, information is power. It's as if there is a hidden political agenda to subvert real data and keep it from coming out publicly. Was the narrative so great that now these parties are embarrassed to upend a story they had sold so well? Or are there villainous forces at play who purposefully steer people in the wrong direction once they get close to the truth? That's the story, and I'm sticking to it... I think it may be a little bit of both. While hospitals were told they would not be getting payments from Medicare unless they toed the line, the physicians who went along with hospital policy for monetary reasons are so embarrassed by their capitulation, since most of their patients know now that they were DEAD wrong!

I wanted to know what percentage of people in the cases that Richard dealt with had these rare clots. Was this an everyday occurrence, or was it rare? I needed to get some perspective on the actual number because that's just my nature, I'm a data guy. Richard pulled out his spreadsheet and started counting, "one, two, four, six, eight, ten, okay, so in this calendar month of April, I see 10 out of 30, so that's 33 percent that had the major stuff, but a lot more of them had clots. Only 4 of the 30 didn't have any clots. However, the number of young people who are dying is increasing." Now, my mind started to go in all different directions because I could envision a spreadsheet to try and build a model to test a hypothesis, but I digress. I wanted to know if there was any way to find out if these patients were "vaccinated", if they had Covid multiple times, or if they had any co-morbidities. There were simply too many directions we could go in to build a model, and I had to come to the realization that I was never going to be able to manage that with limited access to information, but it sure makes you think!

I wanted to get back to the increased occurrences of young people dying, and I needed Richard to put it into some perspective for me. I asked him to explain. "When I was an apprentice back in 2000," he began, "we had a young man who was probably in his early teens. He was getting ready for church and fell over dead. It was totally unexpected. I say that because those cases are so rare that it sticks out in my memory. That young man was born with a congenital heart defect and his family knew that this could happen one day. Then again, in 2005 or 2006, we had a young man who was the spitting image of health. He stepped out of the shower and dropped dead. Again, he had a defect. Now, I can't tell you how many young people I've done lately because it's becoming more and more common. I'm seeing young people like teenagers and children that are dying of cancer, and I can't help but ask myself, is this related to the vaccine?"

I think Richard is asking the same question that all of us have subconsciously thought about, and now, more commonly, consciously ask. When a young football player just stops and falls over on the field of play or when an athlete makes the news in their 20s or 30s because of a death or serious health issues, most of us want to know... Were they vaccinated? Richard brought up an interesting discussion about another young person he saw on his table. He was attending to a young person who had died of cancer, and he found the subject was full of these strange clots. The family stated that the young person was not vaccinated, but Richard was perplexed because every one of the clients he'd had with these strange clots had been "vaccinated" for COVID-19. However, in this instance, Richard thought maybe there was something wrong with the blood supply. Richard stated, "I wondered if she'd had some kind of blood transfusion." Well, about a day later, the funeral director called the family back and asked what kind of treatments she had undergone. Had she been given any blood transfusions?" It turns out that she did indeed have some transfusions about four months prior to her passing.

Richard's data indicated that these fibrous clots, in most instances, were appearing roughly four to five months after receiving their "shots", which puts a rough timeline on their formation. At the time of writing, Richard estimated that about 50 percent of his cases had these clots, which in my mind is a staggering number. The cause and correlation between the timeline of the shots and the percentages of people with these clots, coinciding with the fact that most, if not all, had received the COVID-19 shots, paints a very dark and convincing picture.

Richard put it further into perspective like this, he said, "Let me give you a good analogy, prior to 2021, I would estimate we'd see clotting issues in the deceased about 15 to 20 percent of the time. Some embalmers say around 30 percent of the bodies have some type of clotting. Now, we're talking traditional, jelly-like clots, which can happen when the blood stops moving. I'm not saying that doesn't happen, it happens, and we are very familiar with it. In today's world, I'm lucky to get 15 percent of the bodies that don't have any clots. It is a 180 degrees turn from the way it used to be. So about roughly

85 percent of the bodies have some form of clotting and about 50 percent of those are the white fiber stuff." Those numbers really sunk in.

I see a lot of myself when I talk to Richard. The naysayers want to cry foul and call you every name in the book, but the fact is, they just don't have any data of their own to back up their negativity. When I wrote *Fauci's Fiction*, I just wanted to tell the story of our data. Our story didn't match the whole of the narrative being perpetuated by the governments around the world, big tech, and the mainstream media, but it was solid, and slowly but surely, the masses are catching up. When I talk to Richard, I can hear the frustration, the concern, and the passion in his voice for not only what he does as a profession but for his concern for humanity. He's been figuratively beat up and put through the ringer, all for trying to sound an alarm and get the truth out into the light. He's been ridiculed and questioned because his story wasn't the story that everyone needed to keep a lid on what just may be a nefarious intent. Richard Hirschman doesn't deserve that as a colleague or a professional, and he doesn't deserve that from humanity, which is what he and others are still trying to save.

I truly hope he keeps fighting for the truth and continues his good work. I always say, "We're like those who tried to tell you the earth was round, and you decided to burn us at the stake, then laughed about it a hundred years later." Richard Hirschman deserves a medal for sticking his neck out. I'm sure he'd turn it down and say he was just doing his job, but I hope it doesn't take a hundred years for people to learn from his example. I also hope it doesn't take the same amount of time to start learning from all his valuable experience!

8

HOW DOES MRNA WORK?

FIRST, I WANT TO CLARIFY THAT I am not advocating for or against the use of mRNA technology. Yes, I believe it's mass use during the COVID-19 pandemic was one of the most ridiculous and irresponsible things I have ever seen in my career. Its rollout, all at once, was one giant experiment on the whole of humanity. However, I think it would benefit you to know what this technology is and how it works. The tech may have some very promising benefits and future uses, and it's important to understand how it could benefit humanity moving forward.

An Introduction to mRNA Technology

Messenger RNA (mRNA) technology represents a revolutionary approach in biotechnology and medicine, fundamentally changing how we think about vaccines, gene therapies, and even cancer treatments. Although mRNA technology has existed for decades, its application in medical science has only gained mainstream attention in the past few years, especially with the rapid development of mRNA vaccines during the COVID-19 pandemic. To understand how mRNA technology works, it is essential to grasp its biological underpinnings and how scientists have harnessed this naturally occurring mechanism for therapeutic purposes.

This chapter is a detailed exploration of mRNA technology, covering its biological foundation, how it works, how it was developed, its various applications, and potential future innovations. We will delve into the molecular mechanics of mRNA, how it interacts with the cellular machinery to produce proteins, and how this knowledge has been used to design vaccines and other therapies.

Understanding mRNA: The Basics

To appreciate the scope of mRNA technology, we first need to understand what messenger RNA is and its role in the central dogma of molecular biology. The central dogma describes the flow of genetic information within a biological system, which occurs in three stages: DNA -> RNA -> Protein. In this process, DNA, the repository of genetic information, is transcribed into RNA, which is then translated into proteins, the molecules that carry out various functions within a cell.

1. The Central Dogma of Molecular Biology
DNA (deoxyribonucleic acid) contains the genetic blueprint for building and maintaining an organism. However, DNA is in the nucleus of the cell and cannot directly interact with the protein synthesis machinery located in the cytoplasm. The intermediary between DNA and protein synthesis is RNA (ribonucleic acid).

mRNA is one type of RNA that plays a crucial role in this process. It is a temporary, single-stranded copy of a gene that carries the instructions from DNA to the ribosome, the cellular machinery responsible for protein synthesis. The ribosome reads the mRNA sequence and translates it into a specific protein by assembling amino acids in the correct order, as dictated by the mRNA sequence. This process is known as translation.

2. mRNA Structure

mRNA is a linear molecule composed of ribonucleotides, which include a ribose sugar, a phosphate group, and one of four nitrogenous bases: adenine (A), cytosine (C), guanine (G), or uracil (U) (in contrast to DNA, which uses thymine instead of uracil). The sequence of these bases encodes genetic information, which is read in sets of three bases called codons. Each codon corresponds to a specific amino acid or a stop signal during protein synthesis.

An mRNA molecule consists of several key regions:

- **5' cap:** A modified guanine nucleotide at the beginning (5' end) of the mRNA that protects it from degradation and helps initiate translation.
- **5' untranslated region (UTR):** A region upstream of the coding sequence that helps regulate translation.
- **Coding region:** The portion of the mRNA that contains the codons specifying the sequence of amino acids in the protein.
- **3' untranslated region (UTR):** A region downstream of the coding sequence that influences the stability and localization of the mRNA.
- **Poly-A tail:** A sequence of adenine nucleotides added to the 3' end that stabilizes the mRNA and helps with its export from the nucleus to the cytoplasm.

How mRNA Technology Works

mRNA technology utilizes the natural process of protein synthesis to produce specific proteins for therapeutic purposes. Instead of introducing a foreign protein into the body (as traditional vaccines often do), mRNA technology delivers the genetic instructions for cells to produce the desired protein themselves. This approach has significant advantages in flexibility, speed, and safety compared to conventional therapies and vaccines.

1. The Basic Concept of mRNA-Based Vaccines

An mRNA-based vaccine works by delivering synthetic mRNA that encodes a protein specific to a pathogen, such as a virus or bacterium. Once inside the cell, this mRNA is translated by the ribosomes into the target protein. The immune system recognizes this protein as foreign and mounts an immune response, including the production of antibodies and activation of T-cells. This primes the immune system to recognize and fight the pathogen if it encounters it in the future.

For example, in the case of the Pfizer-BioNTech and Moderna COVID-19 vaccines, the mRNA encodes the spike protein of the SARS-CoV-2 virus. Once the spike protein is produced by the cells, the immune system responds by generating antibodies against it. If the person later becomes infected with the actual virus, their immune system can quickly recognize and neutralize it.

2. Key Components of mRNA Vaccines

To design an effective mRNA-based vaccine, several components need to be carefully engineered:

- **The mRNA sequence:** The core of the vaccine is the mRNA that encodes the target protein. Scientists can design this sequence based on the genetic code of the pathogen. The mRNA must be optimized for stability and efficient translation in human cells.

- **5' cap and Poly-A tail:** Just like naturally occurring mRNA, the synthetic mRNA needs a 5' cap and a poly-A tail to protect it from degradation and ensure efficient translation. Without these modifications, the mRNA would degrade rapidly and be unable to produce enough protein to stimulate an immune response.
- **Lipid nanoparticles (LNPs):** mRNA is a large, negatively charged molecule that cannot easily cross cell membranes. To overcome this challenge, the mRNA is encapsulated in lipid nanoparticles, which are tiny particles made of fats. These nanoparticles protect the mRNA and help it enter the cells. Once inside, the mRNA is released into the cytoplasm, where it can be translated into protein.
- **Stabilizers and adjuvants:** In some cases, vaccines include stabilizers to prolong the shelf life of the mRNA and adjuvants to enhance the immune response. However, mRNA vaccines typically do not require adjuvants, as the mRNA itself and the protein it produces are highly immunogenic.

3. mRNA Uptake and Translation

Once the mRNA is delivered to the target cells, the process of protein production begins. The mRNA is translated by the ribosomes, which read the mRNA's codons and assemble the corresponding amino acids into the target protein. This process occurs in the cytoplasm, outside the nucleus, so the mRNA does not need to enter the cell's nucleus or alter the cell's DNA in any way.

The protein produced by the mRNA is typically identical to the natural protein found in the pathogen. For vaccines, this protein is often a structural component of the virus, such as the spike protein in the case of SARS-CoV-2. Once produced, the protein is displayed on the surface of the cell or released into the bloodstream, where it is recognized by the immune system.

4. Immune System Activation

The presence of a foreign protein triggers an immune response. The immune system recognizes the protein as non-self and begins producing antibodies to neutralize it. Additionally, specialized cells called antigen-presenting cells (APCs) process the protein and present fragments of it to T-cells, which further activate the immune response.

There are two main components of the immune response that are activated by mRNA vaccines:

- **Humoral immunity**: B-cells produce antibodies that can bind to the target protein and neutralize the pathogen.
- **Cell-mediated immunity**: T-cells, particularly cytotoxic T-cells, recognize and destroy infected cells that display the foreign protein.

This dual immune response provides robust protection against the pathogen, as the immune system is primed to respond quickly if the person is exposed to the actual virus or bacterium in the future.

Advantages of mRNA Technology

The use of mRNA in vaccines and therapeutics offers several key advantages over traditional approaches:

1. Rapid Development

One of the most significant advantages of mRNA technology is the speed with which vaccines can be developed. Traditional vaccines, such as those based on inactivated or live-attenuated viruses, require the pathogen to be grown in large quantities in cell cultures or eggs, a time-consuming process. In contrast, mRNA vaccines can be designed and synthesized relatively quickly once the genetic sequence of the pathogen is known.

For example, during the COVID-19 pandemic, scientists were able to develop mRNA vaccines within weeks of identifying the SARS-CoV-2 virus. This rapid response was critical in controlling the spread of the virus and saving lives.

2. Flexibility and Customization

mRNA technology is highly versatile and can be easily adapted to target different pathogens. Once the basic platform is established, new mRNA sequences can be designed for different diseases by simply changing the coding region of the mRNA. This flexibility makes mRNA vaccines an attractive option for emerging infectious diseases, as they can be quickly adapted to respond to new threats.

Additionally, mRNA technology allows for the design of multivalent vaccines that can target multiple pathogens or multiple variants of a single pathogen in a single formulation. This could potentially reduce the number of vaccinations needed to protect against a variety of diseases.

3. No Risk of Infection
Unlike vaccines that use live-attenuated or inactivated viruses, mRNA vaccines do not carry the risk of causing infection. The mRNA only instructs cells to produce a specific protein from the pathogen, not the entire virus or bacterium. Therefore, there is no possibility of the vaccine causing the disease it is designed to prevent.

4. Strong Immune Response
mRNA vaccines have been shown to elicit a strong immune response, often comparable to or better than traditional vaccines. The mRNA itself is recognized by the immune system as a foreign substance, stimulating an innate immune response. Furthermore, the protein encoded by the mRNA is also recognized as foreign, triggering a robust adaptive immune response, including both antibody production and T-cell activation. This comprehensive immune activation ensures a more effective defense against the pathogen upon future exposure.

Challenges of mRNA Technology
Despite its numerous advantages, mRNA technology is not without challenges. Overcoming these barriers has been a significant focus of research and development in recent years.

1. Stability and Storage
One of the major challenges with mRNA is its inherent instability. mRNA is prone to degradation by enzymes called ribonucleases (RNases), which are abundant in the body and environment. This susceptibility to degradation makes it difficult to store and transport mRNA vaccines and therapeutics. For instance, the initial COVID-19 mRNA vaccines from Pfizer-BioNTech required

storage at ultra-low temperatures (-70°C), which posed logistical challenges, particularly in regions without advanced cold chain infrastructure.

To address this, scientists have been working on developing more stable formulations of mRNA that do not require such extreme storage conditions. Advances in lipid nanoparticle technology and modifications to the mRNA sequence have already led to more stable versions of mRNA vaccines that can be stored at standard refrigerator temperatures, although further improvements are still needed.

2. Delivery

Delivering mRNA into cells efficiently is another significant challenge. As a large and negatively charged molecule, mRNA cannot easily cross the cell membrane on its own. This is where lipid nanoparticles (LNPs) come into play. LNPs protect the mRNA from degradation and help it enter cells. However, the delivery efficiency and safety of these nanoparticles need to be optimized, particularly for different tissues and cell types.

Research is ongoing to develop more targeted delivery systems, which could allow mRNA to be delivered directly to specific tissues, such as the liver or immune cells, minimizing side effects and improving therapeutic outcomes.

3. Immunogenicity

While the immunogenic nature of mRNA is beneficial in the context of vaccines, it can pose a challenge in therapeutic applications, such as gene therapies or treatments for chronic diseases. In some cases, the immune system may react too strongly to the introduced mRNA, leading to inflammation or other adverse effects. To mitigate this, researchers are exploring ways to fine-tune the immune response, either by modifying the mRNA sequence to make it less immunogenic or by developing delivery systems that reduce immune activation.

Applications of mRNA Technology

The success of mRNA technology in COVID-19 vaccines has opened the door to a wide range of potential applications beyond infectious disease vaccines. Here are some of the most promising areas where mRNA technology is being explored:

1. Infectious Disease Vaccines

The most well-known application of mRNA technology is in the development of vaccines for infectious diseases. In addition to the COVID-19 vaccines, researchers are working on mRNA vaccines for other viral diseases, such as influenza, Zika, and HIV. The ability to rapidly design and test mRNA vaccines makes this technology ideal for responding to outbreaks of emerging infectious diseases.

2. Cancer Immunotherapy

One of the most exciting areas of mRNA research is its application in cancer immunotherapy. In cancer, the immune system often fails to recognize tumor cells as foreign, allowing the cancer to grow unchecked. mRNA vaccines can be used to teach the immune system to recognize and attack cancer cells by delivering mRNA that encodes tumor-specific antigens. These antigens stimulate an immune response against cancer, potentially shrinking tumors and preventing metastasis.

Several clinical trials are currently underway to test the efficacy of mRNA-based cancer vaccines, with promising early results. Personalized cancer vaccines, which are tailored to the unique mutations in a patient's tumor, are also being developed using mRNA technology.

3. Gene Therapy

mRNA can be used as a therapeutic tool for genetic diseases caused by defective or missing proteins. Instead of introducing a new gene into a patient's cells (as is done in traditional gene therapy), mRNA therapy provides the instructions for cells to produce the missing or defective protein. This approach avoids some of the risks associated with gene therapy, such as insertional mutagenesis (when a new gene disrupts normal gene function), and can be administered repeatedly as needed.

For example, mRNA therapies are being developed for diseases like cystic fibrosis, where a genetic mutation results in the absence of a functional protein. By delivering mRNA encoding the correct version of the protein, the therapy can restore normal function.

4. Autoimmune Diseases and Allergies

mRNA technology also holds promise for treating autoimmune diseases and allergies by inducing immune tolerance. In autoimmune diseases, the immune system mistakenly attacks the body's own tissues. mRNA therapy could potentially "re-educate" the immune system by delivering mRNA that encodes self-proteins, thereby reducing the autoimmune response. Similarly, mRNA could be used to treat allergies by delivering mRNA encoding the allergens, in a form that induces tolerance rather than an allergic response.

The Future of mRNA Technology

As research and development in mRNA technology continue to advance, the possibilities for its application seem almost limitless. Several key areas of future development are likely to shape the next generation of mRNA-based therapeutics:

1. mRNA Design Optimization

One area of focus is optimizing the design of mRNA molecules to improve their stability, translation efficiency, and immune response. Modifying the nucleotide sequence, optimizing codon usage, and incorporating chemically modified nucleotides are some strategies being explored to enhance the therapeutic potential of mRNA. Additionally, improving the design of the 5' cap and poly-A tail, as well as the untranslated regions (UTRs), could further enhance the stability and translation efficiency of mRNA in cells.

2. New Delivery Systems

The development of more advanced delivery systems is another critical area of research. While lipid nanoparticles have proven effective for delivering mRNA, there is room for improvement in terms of targeting specific cell types and reducing side effects. Researchers are investigating new materials, such as polymers and peptides, as well as novel nanoparticle designs that could improve delivery efficiency and safety.

One exciting area of exploration is the use of tissue-targeted delivery systems, which could allow mRNA to be delivered to specific organs or cell types. This would be particularly beneficial for diseases that affect specific tissues, such as the liver, lungs, or brain.

3. Therapeutics for Rare Diseases

mRNA technology has the potential to revolutionize the treatment of rare genetic diseases. Many rare diseases are caused by mutations that result in the absence or malfunction of a single protein. With mRNA therapy, it is possible to deliver the correct version of the protein to affected cells, potentially reversing the disease. Since mRNA therapy does not involve permanent changes to the genome, it can be a safer and more flexible option than gene therapy for treating genetic disorders.

4. mRNA Vaccines for Universal Protection
Another exciting possibility is the development of universal vaccines using mRNA technology. For example, researchers are working on a universal flu vaccine that would protect against all strains of the influenza virus, eliminating the need for annual flu shots. Similarly, mRNA technology could be used to develop vaccines that provide broad protection against multiple coronaviruses, potentially preventing future pandemics.

Conclusion

mRNA technology represents a groundbreaking advancement in biotechnology and medicine, with far-reaching implications for the future of vaccines and therapeutics. By leveraging the natural process of protein synthesis, mRNA technology allows scientists to design and produce vaccines and therapies that are faster, safer, and more flexible than traditional approaches. While challenges remain, particularly in terms of stability, delivery, and immune response regulation, ongoing research and innovation are rapidly addressing these issues.

As research continues to evolve, mRNA-based therapies are likely to play a pivotal role in treating a wide range of diseases, from infectious diseases and cancer to genetic disorders and autoimmune conditions. With its vast potential for customization and rapid development, mRNA technology is poised to revolutionize medicine and improve global health for generations to come.

While mRNA technology offers many advantages, it also presents some significant challenges and limitations. Here are some of the main cons of mRNA technology:

Instability of mRNA

Short-lived nature: One of the biggest challenges with mRNA is its inherent instability. mRNA molecules are highly susceptible to degradation by enzymes called ribonucleases (RNases), which are abundant in the body and in the environment. This means that mRNA-based vaccines and therapeutics need to be carefully formulated to ensure stability.

- **Storage and distribution challenges:** Because of its instability, mRNA vaccines (such as the Pfizer-BioNTech COVID-19 vaccine) initially required storage at ultra-low temperatures (-70°C), making logistics difficult, especially in regions without advanced cold-chain infrastructure. Although newer formulations have allowed for more flexible storage conditions, this remains a logistical issue for mass distribution.

2. Delivery Challenges

Efficient delivery to cells: mRNA is a large, negatively charged molecule that cannot easily pass through cell membranes. To deliver it into cells, lipid nanoparticles (LNPs) are commonly used. While LNPs protect the mRNA and help it enter cells, optimizing these delivery systems is a constant challenge. The efficiency of delivery, tissue targeting, and minimizing potential side effects are areas where further improvement is needed.

- **Adverse reactions to delivery systems:** In some cases, the lipid nanoparticles used to deliver mRNA can cause adverse reactions, such as local inflammation at the injection site or, in rare cases, allergic reactions. These responses are partly due to the immune system reacting to the delivery vehicle rather than the mRNA itself.

3. Immune Overactivation and Side Effects

Innate immune activation: mRNA is recognized by the immune system as foreign material. While this property can help activate a strong immune response in vaccines, it can also trigger excessive inflammation in certain cases. In therapeutic applications (e.g., treating genetic disorders), excessive immune activation could be problematic, causing side effects like fever, fatigue, or more severe inflammatory responses.

- **Potential for adverse reactions:** While mRNA vaccines have been shown to be safe for most people, there have been rare cases of adverse events, such as myocarditis (inflammation of the heart muscle) and pericarditis (inflammation of the lining around the heart), particularly in younger individuals. Monitoring and understanding the mechanisms behind these reactions is an ongoing area of research.

4. Limited Long-Term Data

Novel technology: Despite the decades of research that underpin mRNA technology, its widespread clinical use (especially in vaccines) is relatively new. As such, there is still limited long-term data on its safety and efficacy, particularly for vaccines and therapies used over extended periods.

- **Unknown long-term effects**:** While no significant long-term side effects have been observed in mRNA vaccines so far, their long-term impacts are still unknown, particularly for certain groups (e.g., children, pregnant women). Ongoing studies will help to answer these questions in the future.

5. High Production Costs

Manufacturing complexity: While mRNA technology allows for faster design and development of vaccines and therapeutics, producing mRNA at scale is still complex and expensive. The synthesis of high-quality mRNA, the formulation of stable lipid nanoparticles, and ensuring consistency across batches are all processes that require sophisticated technology and expertise. This can drive up production costs compared to more traditional approaches.

- **Costs for low-resource settings:** The high production and storage costs of mRNA-based products may pose barriers to access in low and middle-income countries, where healthcare systems may lack the infrastructure for widespread distribution of these products.

6. Narrow Window for Protein Expression

Temporary effect: mRNA-based therapies only result in temporary protein production. This can be a limitation in cases where long-lasting effects are needed, such as in treating chronic diseases or genetic disorders. For certain applications, the need for repeated dosing or more frequent administration of mRNA-based treatments might be required, potentially leading to compliance issues or higher costs.

7. Lack of Targeting Specificity

Non-targeted delivery: Current mRNA delivery systems generally deliver the mRNA indiscriminately to a wide range of cells, regardless of where the therapeutic protein is most needed. For example, in gene therapy, it may be critical to target a specific tissue, such as the liver or lungs, and ensure that other tissues are not affected. While research is ongoing to develop more targeted delivery systems, this remains a significant challenge.

8. Vaccine Hesitancy and Public Perception

Misinformation and mistrust: Despite the success of mRNA vaccines in controlling the COVID-19 pandemic, misinformation and skepticism surrounding vaccines in general—and mRNA vaccines in particular—pose a significant barrier to widespread adoption. Concerns over new technology, misconceptions about genetic modification, and fears of long-term side effects contribute to vaccine hesitancy in certain populations.

- **Communication challenges:** Effectively communicating the safety and efficacy of mRNA-based vaccines to the public, while addressing concerns and dispelling myths, remains a challenge for public health officials and scientists.

9. Scalability Issues for Therapeutic Use

Therapeutics versus vaccines: While mRNA technology has shown success in vaccines, scaling it for therapeutic purposes, such as treating chronic diseases or genetic disorders, presents additional hurdles. For some diseases, continuous or repeated administration of mRNA might be required, which could introduce long-term safety concerns or practical challenges in sustained treatment.

- **Personalized treatments:** mRNA technology has potential applications in personalized medicine, such as in cancer immunotherapy, where mRNA is tailored to an individual's tumor profile. However, personalized treatments are expensive and logistically challenging to scale, and they require a high degree of customization that limits their use in broader populations.

Conclusion

mRNA technology has ushered in a new era in medicine, with groundbreaking applications in vaccines and therapeutics. However, it is not without its challenges. Issues like stability, delivery, immune overactivation, cost, and public perception present significant hurdles that need to be addressed to unlock the full potential of mRNA-based treatments. As research continues to evolve, scientists and industry experts are working on solutions to these problems, with the goal of making mRNA technology more accessible, effective, and safe for a wide range of diseases and patient populations.

9

WHAT THE DATA TELLS US!

IT'S EASY TO TELL ANECDOTAL STORIES to illustrate what practitioners are seeing at ground level, but the metrics speak for themselves. Now that you know how VAERS works, and how the metrics make it into the system, it would benefit you to take a good look at what the data tells us. The following chart measures reports of miscarriages and stillborn births related to ALL vaccines since 1990. As you can see, the average was well under 100 per year from 1990 to 2020. In 2021, that number skyrocketed to almost 3,500 and continued to be abnormally high throughout 2022. Emergency use of the COVID-19 vaccines was granted to Pfizer on December 10, 2020, and mass vaccinations began just four days later. Moderna was granted

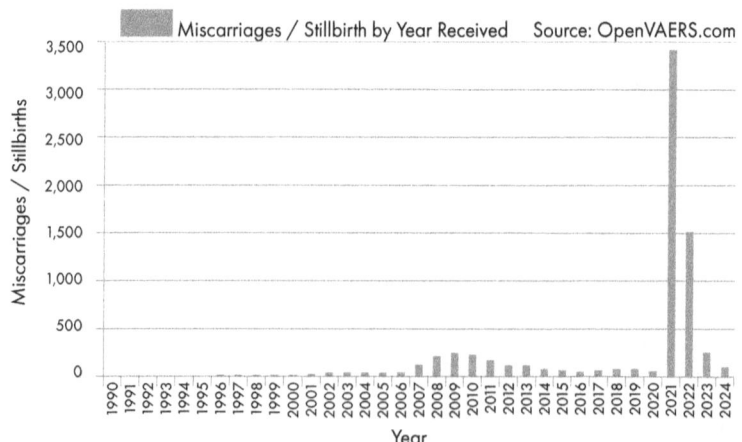

emergency use on December 17, 2020, and Janssen (Johnson and Johnson) was granted emergency use on February 27, 2021. It wasn't until April 19, 2021, that all U.S. states opened eligibility for those 16 and older. Dates for those in other age groups and categories were staggered until August 2021. The point here is that 2021 was the year that these mass "vaccinations" began.

The following chart references menstrual disorders by year. Once again, the data begins in the year 1990 and runs through 2024. As you can see, the numbers are relatively low for a 30-year period until they spike in 2021. They subside slightly in 2022, but are still far above average during the years 2023-2024.

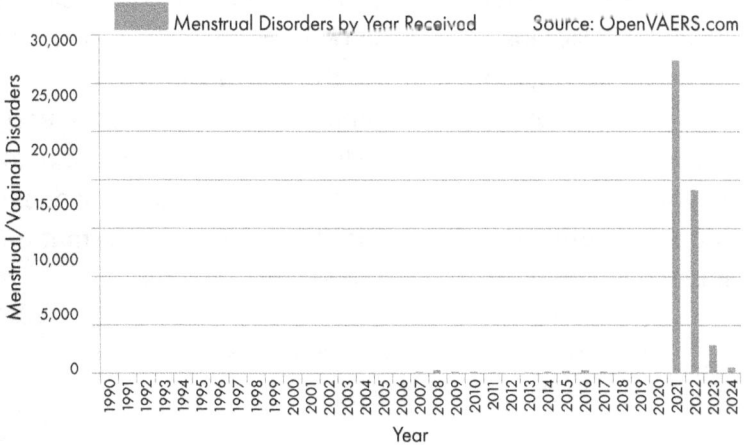

Anaphylaxis is always a concern when administering vaccines. Anaphylaxis is a severe, life-threatening allergic reaction that affects the entire body. When a patient receives a shot in one of our offices, they will wait for 15 minutes to make sure there isn't an allergic reaction before we clear them to leave. While this is rare, it does occur. The following chart highlights anaphylaxis versus severe allergic reaction by manufacturer, by sex, and by age. The smaller values to the left in each graph are anaphylaxis and the larger values are severe. As you can see here, Pfizer is the biggest culprit, with Moderna, Johnson and Johnson, and Novavax trailing behind. It's important to note that we would have to analyze the data of those doses administered by the manufacturer to make sure our data isn't skewed. In other words, if 95 percent of the U.S. population received Pfizer doses, the numbers represented in these charts would naturally be higher because we are cherry picking data in quantity. However, this isn't the case. As of the latest data on COVID-19 vaccinations in the U.S., the distribution of vaccine types is heavily skewed toward mRNA vaccines, specifically, Pfizer-BioNTech and Moderna. The Pfizer-BioNTech vaccine accounts for approximately 48% of the administered doses, while Moderna follows closely with about 42%. Janssen (Johnson & Johnson) makes up a much smaller portion, at around 10% of the total doses given.

Pfizer and Moderna dominate because of their early approval and broader availability, particularly for booster campaigns. Janssen's usage has declined significantly due to concerns about side effects and the single-dose format not aligning with evolving booster recommendations.

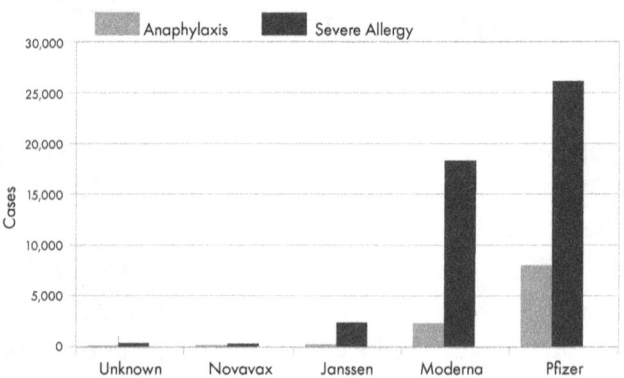
Anaphylaxis Cases Post Covid Vaccine by Manufacturer

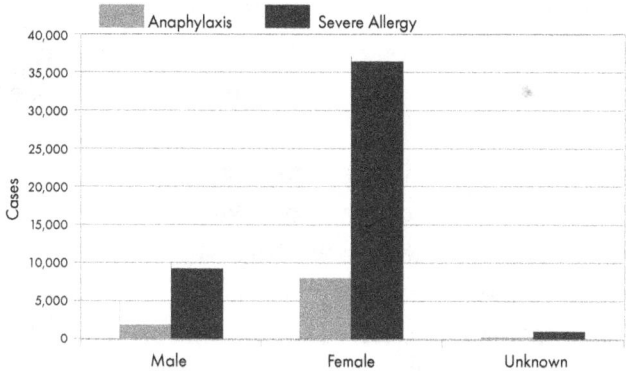

Anaphylaxis Cases Post Covid Vaccine by Sex

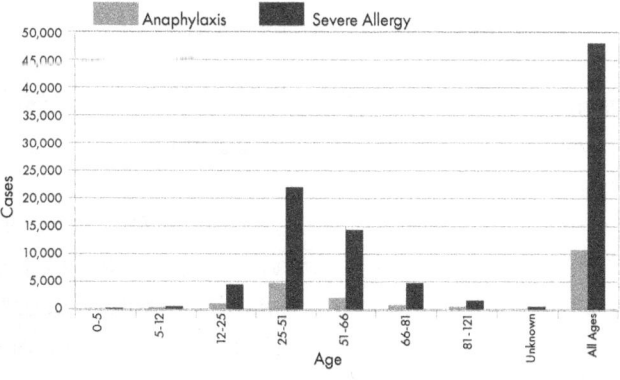

Anaphylaxis Cases Post Covid Vaccine by Age

On another note, I think it's relevant to put the Novavax vaccine into context. I say this because most of what is represented in these charts proves my hypothesis from testing and acquiring data shortly after the vaccines were released. Our initial estimates were that the recipients of these shots would see a higher instance of medical issues from the mRNA technology. When pressed early on about the vaccines, we never recommended any of them because they were unnecessary and did not work as advertised. However, when pressed further about which one was going to do less damage by patients who were steadfast on receiving them, our hypothesis suggested the Janssen shot. Our office only had three types at our disposal, and those were Pfizer, Moderna, and the Janssen shot from Johnson and Johnson. The reason we gravitated towards Johnson and Johnson was because they used traditional and proven technologies. I do want to make it clear that we NEVER recommended any of these shots based on our overwhelming data. If a patient was adamant about receiving a dose and asked for a recommendation, we suggested Johnson and Johnson. However, overall, we NEVER recommended any of these shots. It was only after much pushback from the patient, who were absolutely convinced by the government rhetoric that they needed one, and asked which we recommended out of the three we had that we would make such a recommendation.

Novavax uses another traditional, protein-based technology. Novavax is a protein subunit vaccine. This means it is a protein adjuvant, which is very different from the mRNA technology which was being used en masse. The Janssen shot (Johnson and Johnson) uses viral vector technology, which has also been around a bit longer and has had some successes. To further put this into perspective, when you look at the percentages of the mRNA doses given, you will see a large disparity between the number of cases reported, with Pfizer topping that list. This leads back to Dr. Janci Lindsay's hypothesis that the purest form of this "vaccine" was the worst. Dr. Lindsay stated that when the shot was given in its purest form and not muddied down by different freezer temperatures or transport, these shots would be more harmful. The metrics in all the charts support exactly that.

One of the strange things we saw very early on, which was confirmed in consultation with other providers, was the high number of cases coming into offices with shingles. This was happening at an alarming rate, and in very young people as well. The following chart highlights shingles cases post Covid vaccine by manufacturer, then by sex, and finally by age. As you can see, Pfizer tops the list again with a propensity for women and the age group of 25-51 standing out.

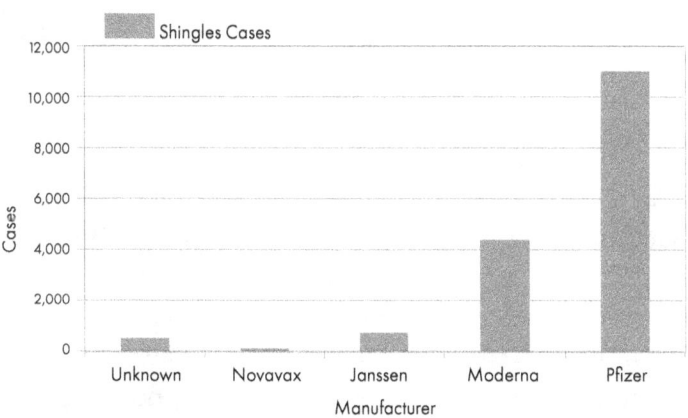

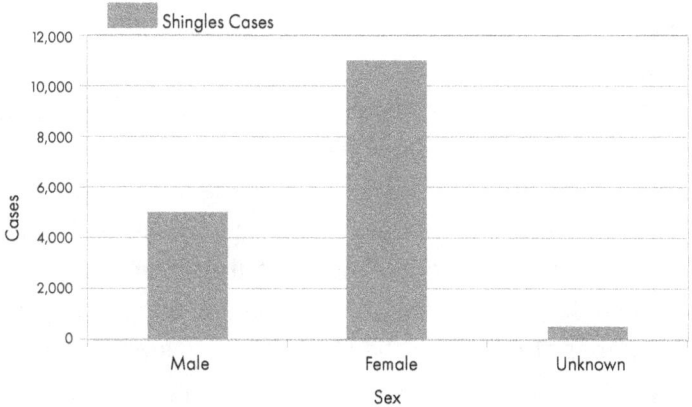

Shingles Cases Post Covid Vaccine by Age

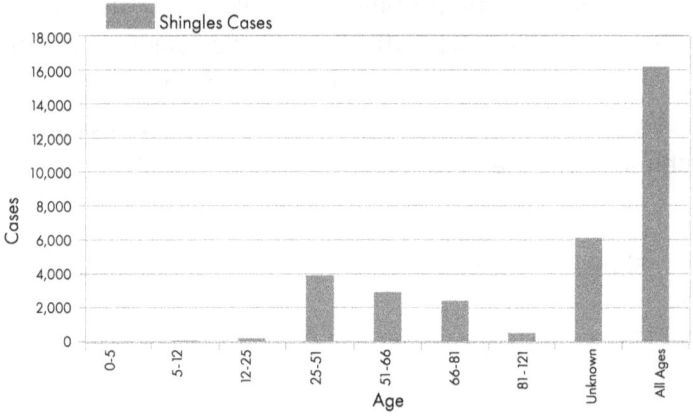

One of the things that's made it into the public forum is the discussion of pericarditis (the inflammation in the sack surrounding the heart) or myocarditis (inflammation of the heart muscle itself). The following chart illustrates the cases of both pericarditis and myocarditis reported for all vaccines. As you can see, the numbers reported were virtually non-existent until 2021, when the values spiked to almost 16,000 cases. Those cases have slowly come down, but to reiterate the perspective here, in 2021, 75 percent of the population was considered "fully vaccinated", while in early 2024, those numbers dropped to about 18 percent.

To put this further into perspective, the following chart represents pericarditis and myocarditis in COVID-19 vaccines versus flu vaccines. This chart groups the number of cases by age and includes all years of data. As you see by the barely visible lines at the bottom of the chart, the adverse effects from the flu shots are not enough to cause any concern. However, the number of cases for the Covid shots is staggering, especially in young adults. It is also worth noting that the flu shots

All Myo/Pericarditis Reported to VAERS by Year (all vaccines)

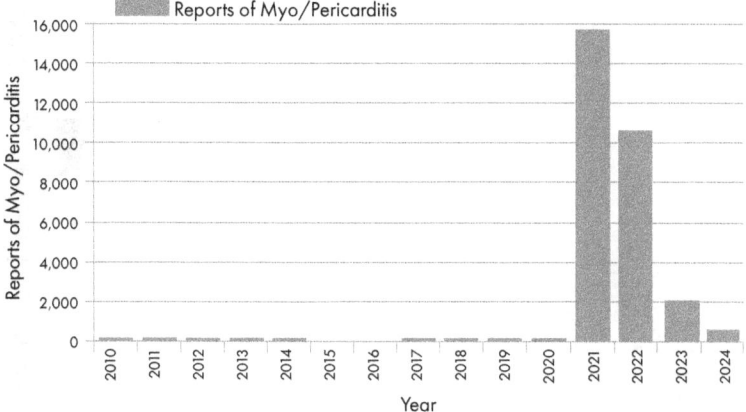

used traditional technology and not mRNA. Additionally, if you read my previous work, reiterated here in *Vaccine Fiction*, I've pointed out many times that it was criminal to call these shots "vaccines". The public's understanding of flu shots compared to a polio vaccine or something similar that would render the patient inoculated was a stretch of the truth that played against common understanding and perception.

Guillain-Barré syndrome is a condition in which the immune system attacks the nerves. The condition may be triggered by an acute bacterial or viral infection. This is why so many practitioners did NOT recommend those Covid shots for patients with this condition. Transverse Myelitis is a rare neurological condition wherein the spinal cord is inflamed. Transverse implies that the spinal inflammation extends horizontally through the cross-section of the spinal cord. Transverse Myelitis can cause paralysis by damaging the spinal cord's myelin sheath, which is the protective coating around the nerve cells. The following chart shows the reporting of both Guillain-Barré and Transverse Myelitis for all vaccines versus flu vaccines from 1990

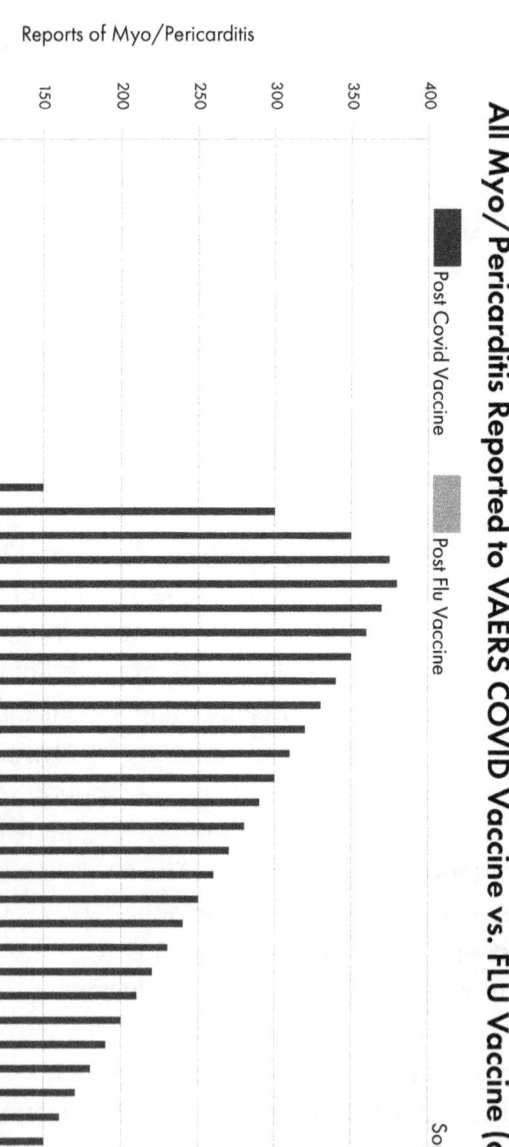

to 2024. While there is always a risk of acquiring one of these syndromes with any vaccination, the numbers in 2021 through 2024 speak for themselves.

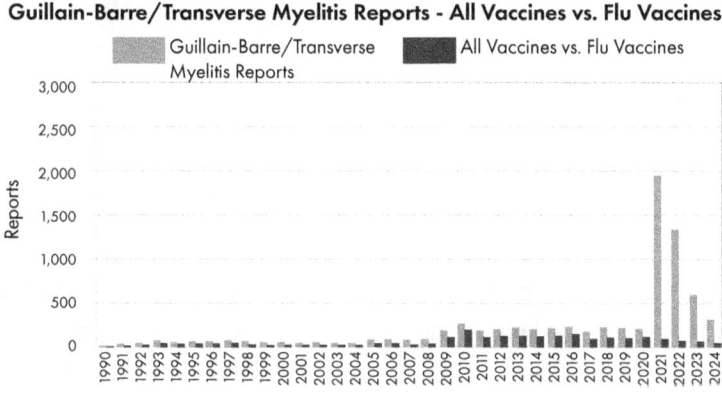

Guillain-Barre/Transverse Myelitis Reports - All Vaccines vs. Flu Vaccines

Myocardial Infarction or a heart attack is a concern for these Covid shots as well. The following chart illustrates the time of a heart attack after "vaccination" onset in days. The second chart illustrates the age groups of those who have reported a heart attack to the VAERS system after receiving a Covid shot.

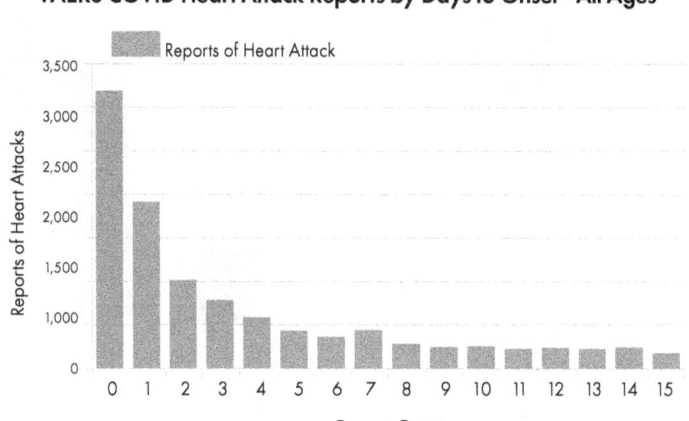

VAERS COVID Heart Attack Reports by Days to Onset - All Ages

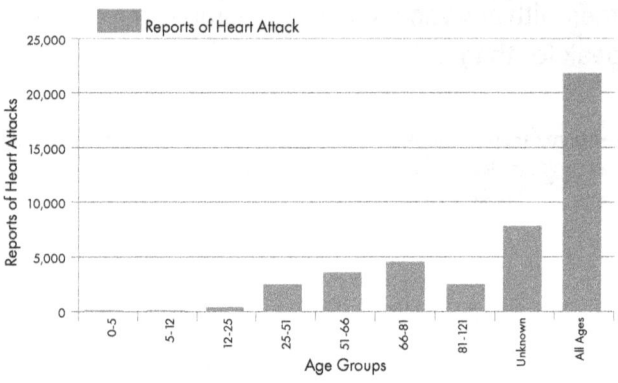

Heart Attack Reports Post Covid Vaccine by Age

There were countless stories of Bell's palsy or idiopathic facial paralysis. This is the sudden weakness in the muscles on one half of the face. Bell's palsy may occur as a reaction to a viral infection and can last upwards of six months. However, it can be permanent due to severe infection that can leave permanent damage to cranial nerve V (5). The following chart illustrates the cases reported to VAERS of Bell's palsy by manufacturer, sex, and finally age group. As you can see, Pfizer takes the cake with a propensity for women, and the age group of 25–51 standing out again.

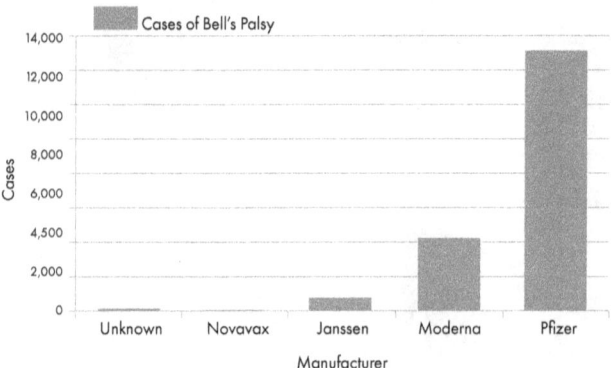

Bell's Palsy Cases Post Covid Vaccine by Manufacturer

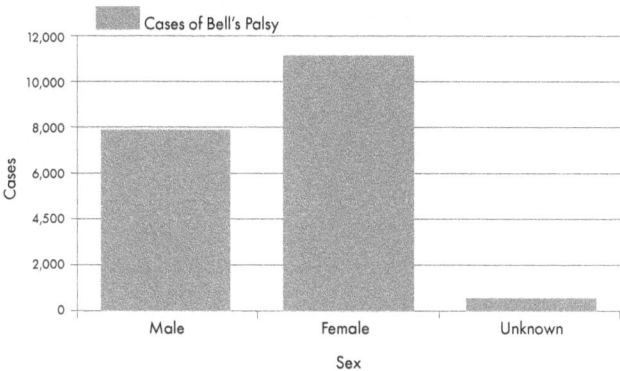

Bell's Palsy Cases Post Covid Vaccine by Sex

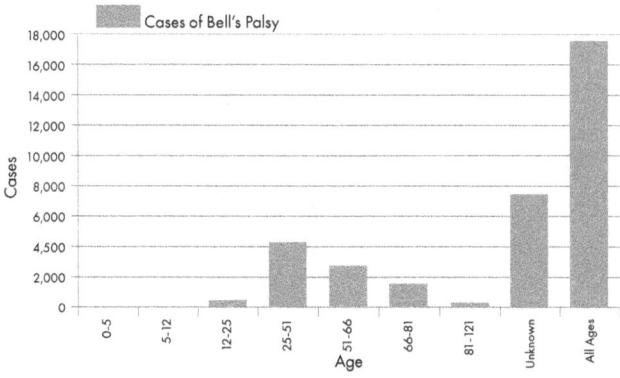

Bell's Palsy Cases Post Covid Vaccine by Age

Thrombocytopenia, or a low platelet level, is also a cause for concern in relation to these Covid shots. Low platelet levels can have causes that aren't due to underlying disease. Examples include pregnancy, altitude, or medication side effects. This condition can cause uncontrolled bleeding and can occur when your immune system makes antibodies that mistakenly identify your cells as being invaders and then direct other immune cells to attack your platelets. The following chart illustrates cases of thrombocytopenia reported to VAERS by manufacturer, sex, and followed by age. Once again, Pfizer tops the list with a

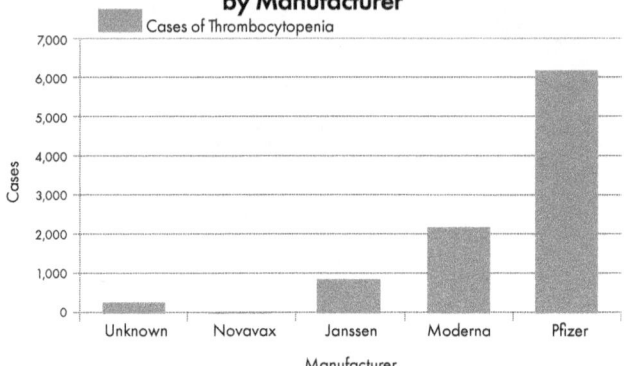

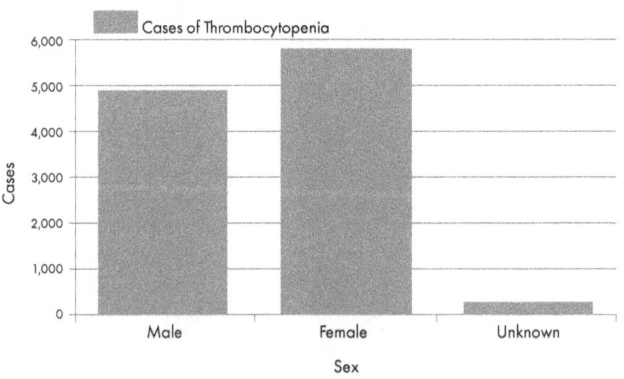

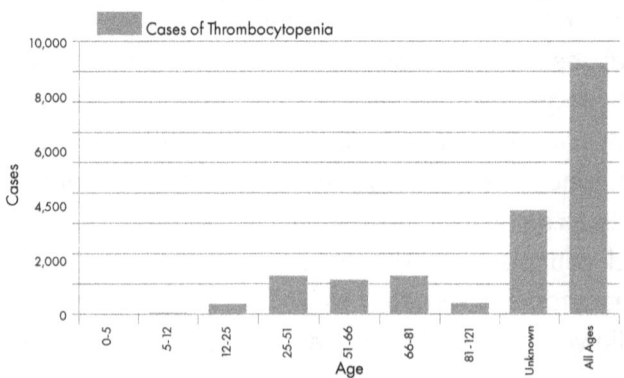

propensity for women, and that age grouping of 25-51 is slightly higher than the rest.

We've all had a visit to the emergency room at one point in our lives or another. The following chart illustrates emergency room visits or urgent care visits reported to VAERS that were specific to COVID-19 "vaccinations" grouped by manufacturer, sex, and then age.

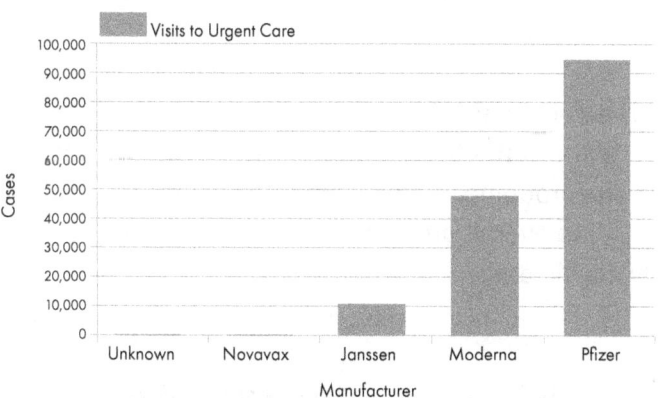

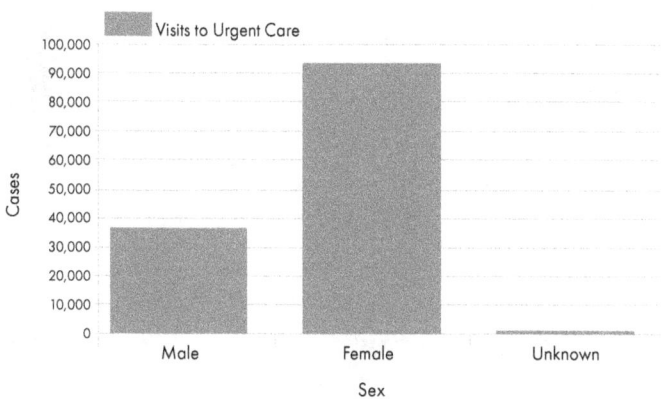

Visits to the ER Post Covid Vaccine by Age

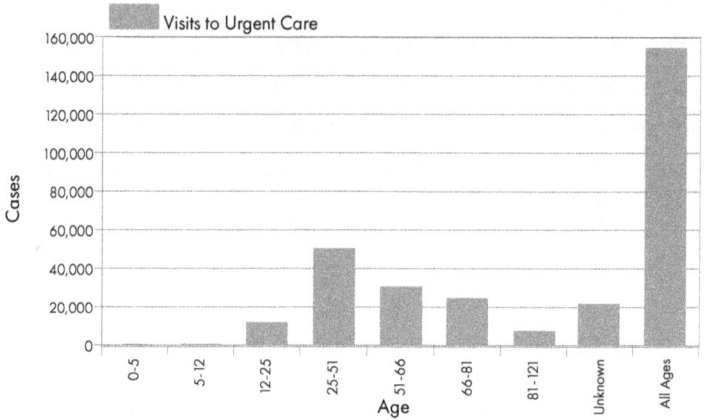

The following chart illustrates a life-threatening event reported into the VAERS system by manufacturer, sex, and then age grouping. While the metric of numbers varies among charts, the overall proportion or ratio they represent remains fairly consistent.

Life Threatening Events Post Covid Vaccine by Manufacturer

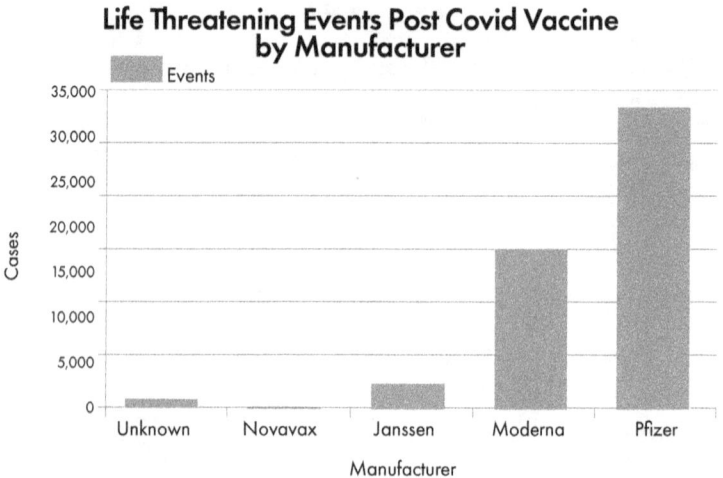

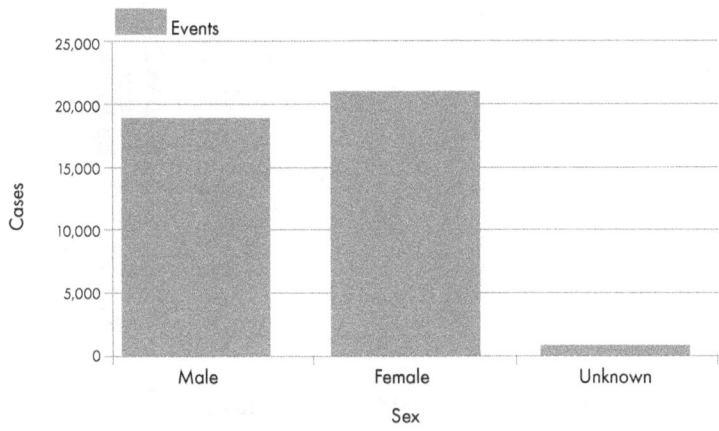

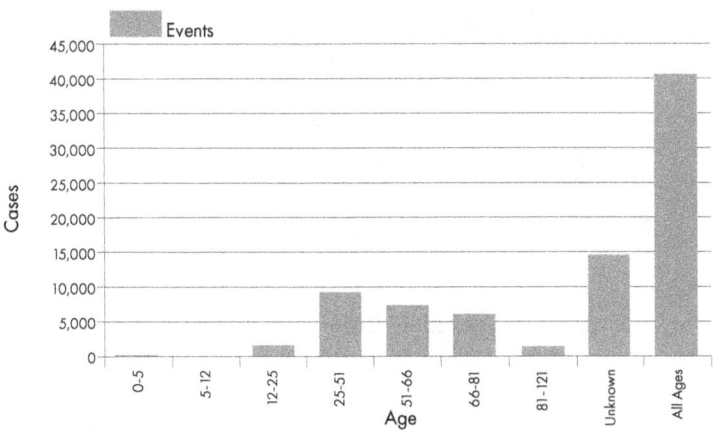

The following chart represents hospitalizations reported due to a Covid shot by manufacturer, sex, and age grouping. I think that by now, you have probably noticed the same trends.

Hospitalizations Post Covid Vaccine by Manufacturer

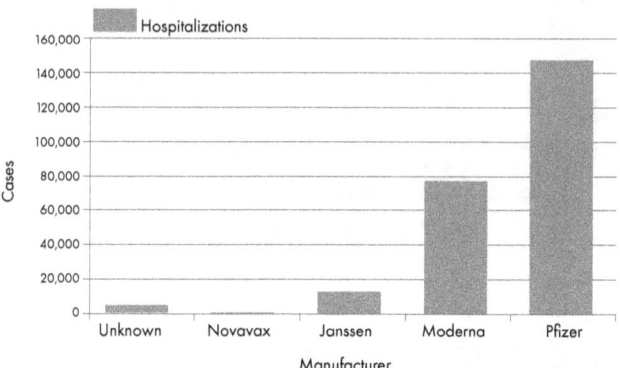

Hospitalizations Post Covid Vaccine by Sex

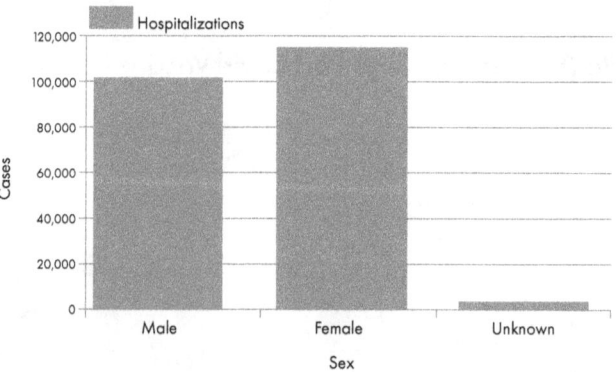

Hospitalizations Post Covid Vaccine by Age

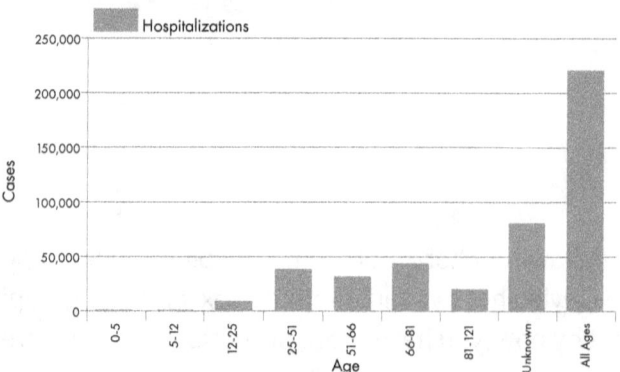

The following chart illustrates a permanent disability reported to VAERS due to a COVID-19 shot. While the metrics may vary, the proportionality remains the same.

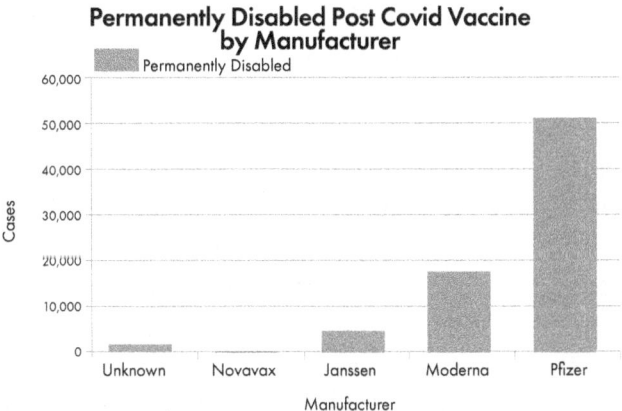

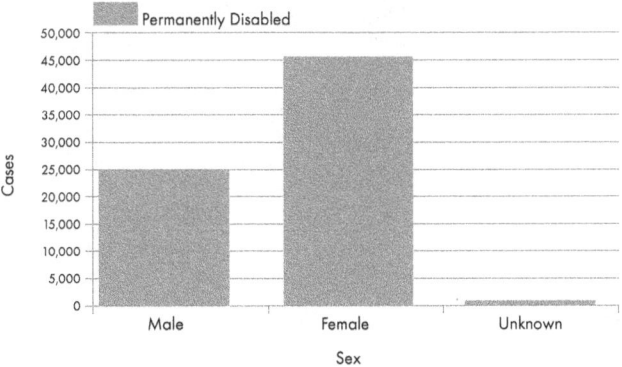

Permanently Disabled Post Covid Vaccine by Age

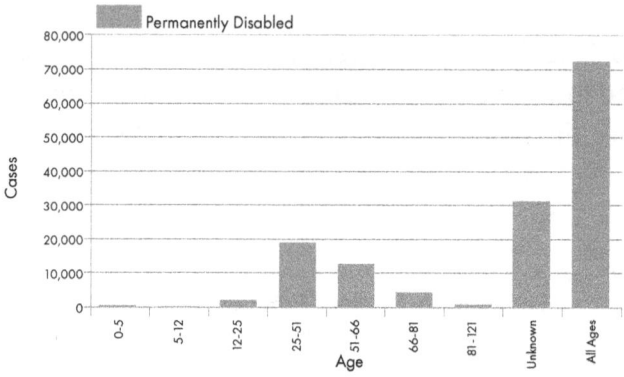

The following chart illustrates the deaths reported to VAERS from all the COVID-19 shots. While the naysayers may look at these numbers and purport a much larger COVID-19 mortality rate, saying that the risk was worth the reward, I will reiterate that most people did not die of COVID-19. Most died early on due to the novelty of the virus and the treatment methods used. We predicted the mortality rate of COVID-19 would be close to or right on par with influenza in April 2020, and those numbers

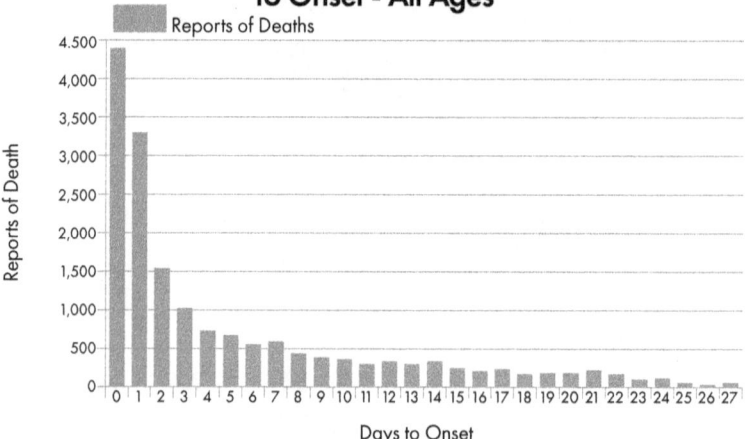

Life Threatening Events Post Covid Vaccine by Sex

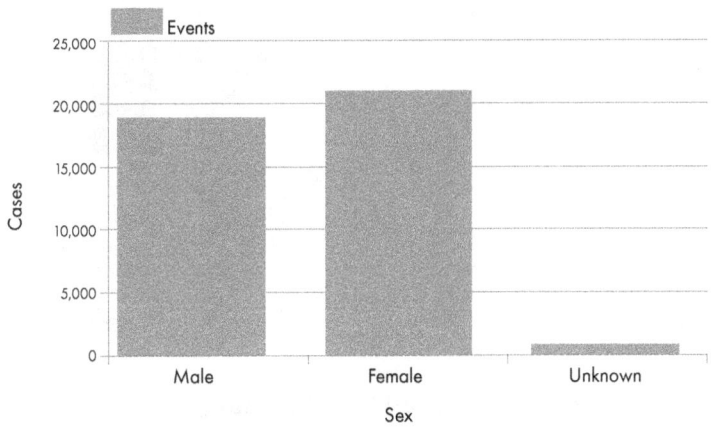

Life Threatening Events Post Covid Vaccine by Age

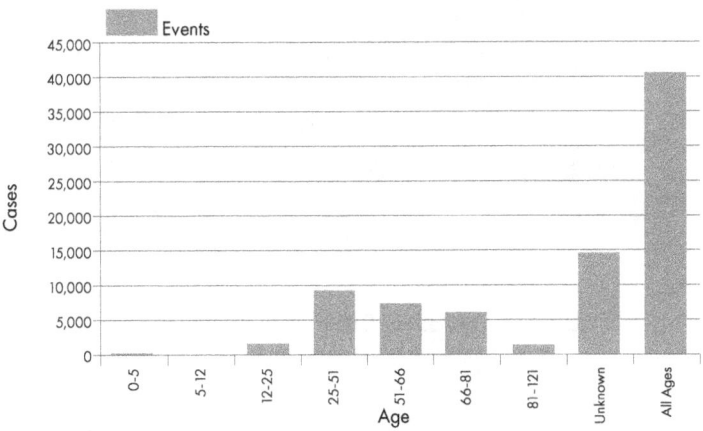

The following chart represents hospitalizations reported due to a Covid shot by manufacturer, sex, and age grouping. I think that by now, you have probably noticed the same trends.

Hospitalizations Post Covid Vaccine by Manufacturer

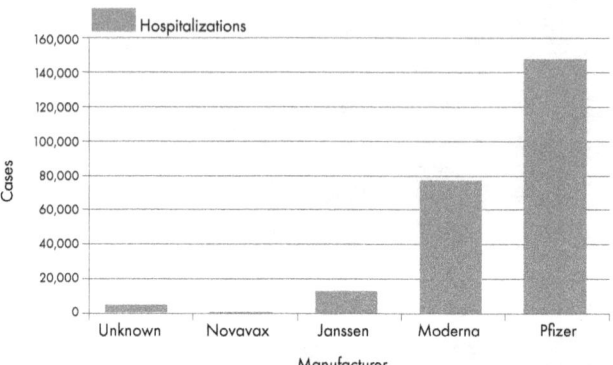

Hospitalizations Post Covid Vaccine by Sex

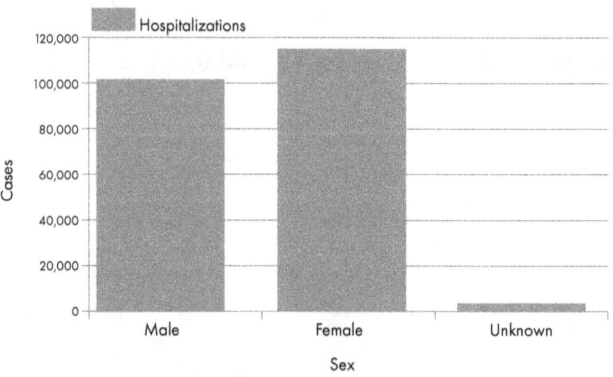

Hospitalizations Post Covid Vaccine by Age

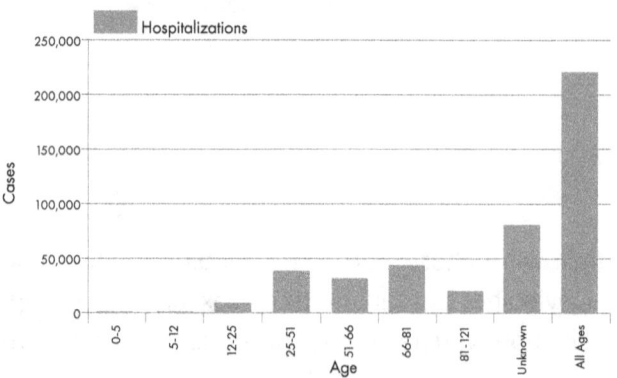

have proven to match now we have had more time to digest the data. The chart below shows deaths after days of onset.

Finally, the last chart illustrates all deaths reported to VAERS by year due to a vaccine. The data ranges from 1990 through 2024, consistent with the other charts in this chapter. The numbers speak for themselves and correlate exactly with the timeframe of the mass rollouts of these "vaccines".

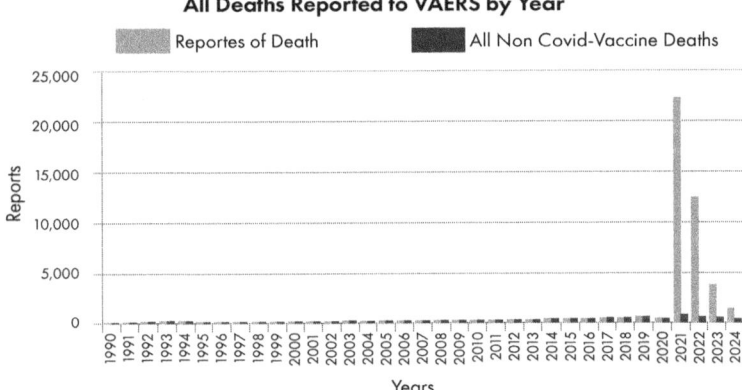

Still, and for some reason, governments and manufacturers are continuing to push the narrative and encourage everyone to run out to get their latest COVID-19 booster. It consistently amazes me that we are still living in this bizarro world for a virus that has the same mortality rate of influenza and still using a shot that doesn't work. The Swine flu vaccination got pulled off the market after 26 deaths from Guillain-Barré, but here, with thousands of deaths related to these Covid shots, particularly the mRNA shots, the public outcry is non-existent. Lastly, if you recall how the VAERS system works, only a very small percentage of data makes it into the system. While these numbers may seem overwhelming, this is just the tip of the iceberg. The true scope of the problem is unfathomable!

10

HOW THE MEDIA IS PORTRAYING THIS

ANYONE WHO'S INVESTIGATED THE COVID-19 PANDEMIC or the efficacy of the Covid "vaccines" can tell you that there is some kind of media bias, that's if they are paying attention. It's very different for a guy like me who's published a book on Covid. I've had an inside look at what happens when forces actively try to ban you, discredit you, and censor your information. I never expected it, but one learns every day, at least I like to try to learn something new every day. What I didn't know was that the lessons were hard fought, and unless you've been through it yourself, they seem downright surreal.

I used to hear people talk all the time about "shadow-banning". I would hear terms like "deep state" and "censorship" and think to myself, in my own idealistic way, "But we live in a free country, with free speech and press!" I thought, even if people were trying to censor something, the media was the fourth estate, the beacon of free speech, surely they would expose whatever lies were being thwarted upon us ordinary citizens... Nope, that's not the way it works, folks. When you are in a battle to uncover the truth, nothing is more frustrating than fighting day in and day out just to get shut down by even the people you thought would have your back.

The media's portrayal of vaccines related to COVID-19 has varied significantly depending on the source, with coverage often influenced by political, scientific, and cultural perspectives. Broadly, mainstream outlets have generally supported the efficacy and safety of COVID-19 vaccines, but seldomly address concerns over rare side effects and vaccine hesitancy.

1. Mainstream Media

In major outlets like The *New York Times*, CNN, and BBC, COVID-19 vaccines were often framed as essential tools in combating the pandemic. Articles emphasized their efficacy in preventing severe illness, hospitalization, and death, particularly as variants like Delta and Omicron emerged. Reports also highlighted scientific consensus on vaccine safety and the rigorous processes vaccines underwent for emergency use approval. Public health experts and doctors were frequently quoted to encourage vaccination and dispel misinformation, while avoiding addressing concerns like myocarditis, blood clots, or other rare side effects that could arise post-vaccination.

2. Alternative Media and Vaccine Skepticism

In contrast, some alternative or conservative media outlets portrayed COVID-19 vaccines more critically. Platforms such as The *Epoch Times*, Fox News, and Natural News focused more heavily on the risks associated with vaccines, often amplifying reports of adverse reactions or questioning government mandates. These sources sometimes highlighted concerns about the speed of vaccine development, the potential for long-term side effects, and the transparency of pharmaceutical companies. Coverage in these outlets was more likely to appeal to vaccine-hesitant or skeptical audiences.

3. Misinformation and Social Media

Social media platforms were flooded with both accurate information and misinformation. Sites like Facebook, Twitter, and YouTube took measures to combat the spread of vaccine misinformation, yet theories—ranging from vaccines altering DNA to causing widespread infertility—were prevalent. However, many of these theories turned out to be correct. These narratives contributed to vaccine hesitancy and sparked debates over freedom of choice versus public health responsibility.

Overall, the media's portrayal of COVID-19 vaccines has been polarized, with mainstream media promoting the benefits and safety of vaccines, while certain outlets and social media channels either raised skepticism or propagated misinformation. The balance between reassuring the public and addressing legitimate concerns continues to shape vaccine-related coverage.

I go back and forth with my publicist on this all the time. She gets it, and she's good, that's why I hired her! Like-minded people always get along, and people feel more comfortable when you know your core group has your best interests in mind. I've done countless TV and radio shows and even more podcasts to promote my work. I'm happy to talk to anyone at any time to get the truth out. In fact, so are a lot of the media hosts I work with. The problem is big tech for the most part. Whenever I do a show, most hosts won't republish the interview on social media, especially YouTube. The YouTube platform is a big money-maker for those hosts monetizing social media. While you may think that getting big numbers for YouTube would be a good thing for the host, the platform has systematically shut down accounts of people even talking about Covid or the shots. Hosts whose largest audience is on YouTube usually won't touch me with a 10-foot pole!

For television stations, the news cycle drives the narrative. Every time news breaks about Dr. Fauci or someone related to the COVID-19 pandemic, I may get a few requests to come on and comment but most of the work we've done gets ignored, and you really can't say too much during a five-minute television segment. Besides the fact that after four years into this, most people are just outright sick of Covid. What I thought was going to be one of the biggest blockbusters of the century turned out to be a dud. I mean, people were locked down, businesses closed, kids were out of school, suicide rates went up, and for those people who died during the pandemic of whatever circumstance, a lot of them couldn't even attend their loved one's services because of draconian restrictions. I thought, for sure, the media would want to talk about this. It would be like if OJ had a taped confession on his deathbed, and we finally got confirmation on what everyone suspected all along...

There are pockets of people who still want to drive the conversation, and I applaud them because analyzing the data we have in an intelligent way can change the course of how we treat viruses, bacteria, and any pathogens moving forward. It could prepare us for the next big one, or should I say, the "real one" when it comes to fruition. It may not happen in my or your lifetime, but it is bound to come calling one day. We have people on the left who will go with the flow and continue to think that everything that was said from the White House podium was gospel, and you have people on the right who've gone down every perceivable rabbit hole to disprove even themselves, after absorbing so much that they turn 180 degrees from their original argument.

The media, on the other hand, is full of people with the same bias, but they are beholden to other masters. It still amazes me when I see a commercial for Pfizer or Moderna on television, now trying to push whatever round of shot is currently out. In fact, now I see more commercials for just about every kind of vaccine known to man, while the hospital systems that used to ask every patient about their vaccination status upon admittance have now suddenly gone quiet, yes, they don't ask that anymore. Maybe they realized these things didn't work and aren't needed, which was exactly what we were telling our own patients before they even came out. The media has gone eerily quiet as well. The only grumblings you hear about Covid are what I mentioned earlier, when a player like Fauci gets in trouble for admitting some of the recommendations they based their directives on Covid weren't based in science whatsoever, or a new study comes out as a counternarrative to what had been touted for such a long time. When you talk about vaccines, most people tell me EXACTLY the same story, "I got the first one and the booster, but I'm not getting any more of them." To which I say, "If you were our patient, you wouldn't have gotten any in the first place!"

When you deal with the censorship all day, every day, you try to find ways around it. You try to get your message out without getting flagged on YouTube or Facebook. To be blunt, if big tech and social media would just get out of the way, most people could come to terms with what we just went through and the shots, but I would be interested to know if YouTube and Facebook forced "vaccinations" on their staff with repercussions like termination for non-compliance. That tells me enough about their bias and what they want out in the public. When I post a video for any of my work, I don't use the words "Fauci's Fiction", "the book on Covid", or any of the terms that seem to trigger a block, ban, shadow-ban, or whatever you want to call it. I leave the books out of sight, and I make sure to use different words other than "vaccine" or "shots". I start to sound like the biggest idiot to those who don't understand that if I'm not careful with my choice of words, my posts just don't get seen. In many cases, I get messages back saying that I "don't comply with their community standards". If you're not in this game and are just posting stories of your latest kid's soccer game or a recipe for chicken masala, you're probably not getting the same scrutiny that I am over a subject that is still highly toxic.

The very first interview I did was on my friend Kato Kaelin's podcast. Kato co-hosts the "One Degree of Scandalous" show with Tom Zenner. We recorded the interview in West Hollywood a few months before my first book came out. I'll never forget Tom telling me to try to not say the word "Covid" or "Vaccine". He said I should try using "jab" or something else because it affects their views. I said, "Really, that much?" Tom said it was like night and day, and social media would bury it. Most of their shows get thousands of views, in some cases hundreds of thousands, so I thought this would be a great opportunity to promote what I was about to release. Even our buddy comedian Tom Mabe was on the episode, and Tom Mabe has a huge following, which could only help bolster the numbers of viewers tuning in... When the show got released, the views were mediocre to say the least, I gave up even looking after a while because after a few weeks, it was stuck at around 300 in total, while the episodes surrounding mine were in the many thousands and some in the millions. That was my first experience in dealing with suppression, throttling down, and shadow-banning of the subject. I felt responsible—Kato was trying to help, and I somehow made his show a dud with this taboo topic.

When you're in the thick of it, you can only hope that times will change, that the powers that control these things will lighten up or loosen their grip on free speech. I hate to report that the same thing still happens today, and with the same rigor and frequency. You are NOT being told the truth if you listen to mainstream media. And you aren't getting the full story if you get your news from social media either! In fact, you're being sold a bill of goods that may be counter to reality, which is kind of like living in the matrix! Sounds crazy, right? I would have thought it was crazy talk too until I started seeing all this firsthand. It's not fun for an author, and it's doubly hard on the public, they just don't know it yet.

Sensationalism drives what the media wants to report on. Most of the outlets know exactly who their audience is, and they cater to them. The outlets that hope to drive conspiracy theories are usually too far down a rabbit hole to want to dissect real science and data. And the outlets that avoid conspiracy theories think that anything counter to the mainstream narrative on Covid *is* a conspiracy theory. Working on Covid, I was always baffled that the doctors at the White House weren't catching up to what we were seeing on the ground. Then, when I wrote a book about it, I was baffled that the mainstream media didn't want to report on it. It took me a bit until I figured out that, basically, they were the same thing. It's going to take years before the public has any clue, and by then, most of us who lived through it will be long gone. It will be something our kids and grandchildren look back on and study in school, just like we look back at our parents who hid under their desks during a nuclear drill. They will look back and say, "What in the hell were they doing?"

There are some great outlets, but we don't get our news from one of three or four sources like we did when I was a kid.

Information comes at us from all directions. While kids tell me they get much of their news from social media, older people still like to tune into the Six O' Clock news. There are literally thousands of news outlets, publications, shows, podcasts, etc., to pick from, and everyone seems to be going in a different direction. It's no wonder people are skeptical when they hear something counter to what they are being fed. It still amazes me, though, that the Covid narrative was so controlled and so orchestrated that there remains a certain segment of the population rushing out to get their latest booster shot. The sad part is, it's mostly the elderly population because they are still glued to those mainstream media sources. Those mainstreams usually have extensive partnerships with Google, YouTube (which is owned by Google) and Meta, which is Facebook and Instagram. So, if you are trying to follow the money, you need to look no further, and if you are trying to get to the bottom of something, they will tell you left is right and up is down just to distract you from what you're looking for.

We started doing a show on Rumble, which touts itself as a free speech platform, and so far so good. Let's just hope it stays that way. For the record, they have never tried to censor anything we've ever produced, and they have been a very easy platform to work with, so I don't foresee anything changing, at least I hope it won't. Our channel, at the time of writing, gets over 1 million views per month, but ultimately, my audience is in the same bubble as I am. It's the people outside that bubble that really need the lesson. The ones on the inside have already been looking for alternatives to the mainstream media and are highly intelligent. We do love our audience, but it's the ones on the outside that need the lesson.

If you read what the media and the World Health Organization have declared as misinformation, the paradox of why the media is portraying information regarding Covid or the "vaccines" in a certain light becomes obvious. One of the things the WHO has declared misinformation is the statement "the virus can be transmitted via the 5G network". While the statement of this being misinformation is correct, they then mix in some questionable things after that. By blending obvious misinformation with items that appear questionable, they make it seem like all that they present is misinformation. Does that make sense? The following sentence is also classified by the WHO as misinformation; "The virus was manually created in a lab by government leaders." The fact is, even the Federal Bureau of Investigation (FBI) has gone on record to say that there is more evidence than not that this was caused by a lab leak in Wuhan, China. To classify something as misinformation is blatantly false when there is no proof it *is* misinformation. The WHO should have come out and said it was "missing information."

I often wonder who the fact-checkers are, since they seem to fact-check my own proprietary data often. They've never reviewed my data, and they've never called me for comment, but they are quick to slap a label on something I post. Sources say that because of "misinformation", several fact-checking websites that utilize information from the CDC and WHO to debunk common viral information have appeared. Newsflash, the Centers for Disease Control and World Health Organization had most of their information wrong the entire time. They are the two organizations that have lost the most amount of trust among the public for their mishandling of the pandemic. Both were wrong on predicted mortality rates, lockdowns, masking, social distancing, etc. If news organizations are reliant on fact checking sites that are in turn reliant on the CDC and WHO, we are all doomed.

Remember Chris Cuomo? Cuomo, a former CNN anchor, recently shared his personal experience with side effects he believes are related to the COVID-19 vaccine. During an interview on his "News Nation" program, Cuomo disclosed that he has been dealing with ongoing health issues, which he attributes to the vaccine he received during the pandemic. He highlighted that discussions about potential side effects have been limited, suggesting that many are reluctant to address these issues openly due to concerns about assigning blame.

Cuomo's current stance contrasts with his earlier views during the height of the pandemic, when he was a strong proponent of vaccination. He had previously emphasized the importance of vaccination as a pathway to returning to normalcy and had supported vaccine mandates. His shift in position and acknowledgment of his own health challenges have drawn considerable attention and criticism, particularly from those who felt targeted by his earlier advocacy for strict COVID-19 policies. He was adamant that the rest of us had lost our minds, and he was steadfast in his position, even without any data of his own! The problem is, even though Cuomo has come out to contradict his initial statements, those statements were what drove a lot of people to get their shots. The damage is done, and he would have been better off saying he was speculating. The very people we trusted to dig into something and do a little vetting for us were the ones who laid down their swords and went along with the narrative. Sorry, Chris, although you finally spoke up, your credibility is ruined, and in turn, you've discredited your new outlet.

Recent media coverage on COVID-19 vaccines has focused on the rollout of updated vaccines for the 2024-2025 season, aimed at new variants like the KP.2 strain. The updated vaccines include formulations from Moderna, Pfizer, and Novavax, each targeting specific strains to better match the variants circulating this season. Public health agencies, like the CDC, recommend these vaccines for everyone aged six months and older to protect against severe illness and hospitalization. Media discussions also emphasize the importance of timing for vaccinations, especially with the rise in cases during late summer and the upcoming fall and winter. The CDC advises people to get vaccinated by mid-October to ensure protection during peak travel and gatherings over the holidays. This was something that lacked credibility early on for us in our offices. I was adamant that these Covid shots work just like flu shots, and always told our patients that people wouldn't just have a flu shot at anytime of the year. They worked best if they received it right before flu season. Yet, the CDC was having people run out and get shot after shot as soon as the updated boosters were available. Sorry, CDC, you had your chance at maintaining your credibility as well, and you blew it.

In addition to effectiveness against current variants, there is also coverage of side effects and safety concerns. Reports continue to evaluate the risk-benefit profile of the vaccines, noting that while side effects such as soreness and mild fever are common, serious adverse events remain rare—at least that's what they tell you. Surveillance continues for potential issues like Guillain-Barré syndrome and other conditions, with studies underway to better understand these risks. Remember, outlets can only report what data remains readily available, but if the data hasn't made it into VAERS and the studies are flawed, the real information never makes it to see the light of day.

Overall, the media narrative around COVID-19 vaccines now balances encouraging uptake of the updated vaccines with addressing concerns and uncertainties about side effects, adapting to evolving data on their efficacy against new variants.

In all, it's too little too late. We knew early on what we needed to communicate to keep ourselves and our neighbors safe. The media chose not to listen when they should have been digging a little deeper and asking the question, "Why are you saying all this?" They discounted our real data in favor of CDC and government narratives. The journalists who want to regain their credibility should do a deep dive into what went wrong, and maybe this time they would have the story of the century.

In April 2020, media coverage of COVID-19 dominated the news cycle, reflecting the peak of the initial global response to the pandemic. During this time, it is estimated that between 40% and 60% of news content across major media outlets was directly related to COVID-19. This included updates on case numbers, government responses, public health measures, and the impact on daily life. In contrast, as of this writing and a little more than four years after the initial outbreak, recent data suggests that now around 1% of articles from high-traffic news sites focus on COVID-19, but these stories still attract a notable share of audience attention, indicating that interest remains when new developments or concerns arise. The tone of coverage has also evolved, with a mix of informative updates about vaccine availability and safety, as well as reports on new variant trends. But the coverage is still lacking the story that needs to be told. What a shame! And what a disservice to the audience—it's almost criminal.

11

BIG PHARMA AND ADVERTISING

I HEAR THAT TRAVIS KELSEY IS PRETTY good at football, but I never knew he had experience with data and healthcare... I guess, for me, watching the continuation of COVID-19 commercials and advertisements is a little different. I mean, my perspective is completely different from the public's, and trying to get them to come around and see what I see has been more challenging than I initially anticipated. But why take my word for it when you can learn everything you need to know from Martha Stewart? Martha was featured in an ad for Pfizer encouraging people to get the new updated COVID-19 booster that was engineered for the Omicron variants in 2023. If I were able to plug Martha into my head for just a moment, she would know that our offices never recommended those Covid shots because they weren't needed. She would also have known that they don't work, and we still didn't have enough data to show that they wouldn't be harmful in the long term.

When I see someone come out and shill for a product that doesn't work or represents a principle that's later proven false, it makes me question everything they say in life. I know Martha was most likely compensated for her participation in that commercial, unless she thought she was doing something to save all of humanity or some self-righteous thing like that. It reminded me of all the celebrities who appeared in commercials for FTX, run by Sam Bankman Fried. When he got caught defrauding all his investors, the celebrities who appeared in all the FTX spots ran for the hills. The problem with the Covid shots is that even though most of the arguments made for them have had hole after hole shot in them, there is a certain segment of the population, government, and dare I say it, special interest groups, that keep patching up those holes to keep their ship afloat, just long enough until nobody really notices it was ever sinking.

It further amazes me that the "almighty dollar" takes precedence over life itself, or at least that's how it seems. When it comes to money, as in Sam Bankman Fried's case, everyone attributes culpability and demands accountability. When it comes to lives being lost from an untested, unproven, and unneeded shot, people seem to look the other way. They shut down and won't even have a conversation about it. They'll angrily say things like, "we just didn't know", until I tell them that my patients were well-informed right from the start. Why does the average citizen want to run cover for the pharmaceutical companies and the media outlets who had this thing wrong from the beginning? There must be some cognitive distortion involved. Maybe that will change when their own doctors come around or when they or someone close to them gets an adverse reaction to one of these shots. Maybe they'll have to catch COVID-19 for the twelfth time to realize that their multiple boosters didn't work and were never going to work!

I wonder if this is because money itself doesn't have a political affiliation, but COVID-19 unfortunately took one on. Either way, cognitive distortion or cognitive dissonance always intrigues me. Since I drew a comparison from COVID-19 to the financial industry, I decided to ask my friend Ralph Johnson, a financial expert, if this was any different in his world and why people in the case of Sam Bankman Fried and FTX may have been more vocal about being taken for a ride. He responded by saying, "It's true, when people lose money, there is a little shame in admitting they were duped. The deciding factor in coming out usually has to do with how much they lost, how much they need it back, how many other people were duped, and how egregious the fraud was. The bigger the numbers on those four items, the bigger the outcry."

That got me thinking a bit. The comparisons are real, but money is always tangible and fungible, health is not. Many people get adverse reactions to these shots long after they've received it, so drawing a correlation between the two doesn't always occur. Also, the ones who haven't gotten a reaction or don't realize that these shots changed something in their health aren't going to come out and participate in the outcry. Besides, big pharma still runs commercials in the mainstream media, so the public is consistently told that they need to "get their booster" or protect others from "new variants". Why would anyone want to go against the grain and put themselves out there? Is the reward bigger than the risk that person would take? As Ralph stated, there are a lot of factors that come into play in whether someone comes out and admits they were duped.

With the pandemic quickly becoming an endemic, Pfizer doubled down in November 2023 by putting all their celebrities into one commercial. Singer John Legend, professional soccer player Megan Rapinoe, singer Charlie Puth, and personalities Martha Stewart and Travis Kelce all appeared in one ad for the company to show unity and diversity among the ranks. The company ran ads with the phrase, "Got yours?", which was reminiscent of the ad campaign for milk back in the 1980s. The celebs showed off their Band-Aids in a plea for the American public to follow suit. One would think that if the shot was that "safe and effective" against a truly deadly virus, the pharmaceutical companies wouldn't have to spend all that money on paid celebrities to try and persuade the public. So why did they? Because sales are down as the masses start to catch up!

The pharmaceutical industry has seen tens of billions of dollars pour into their companies from both the COVID-19 shot as well as the anti-viral drug Paxlovid. However, as people have started to realize that these shots were unnecessary and even dangerous, the sales that were once abundant have all but dried up. In October 2023, Pfizer announced its fiscal results for the third quarter of 2023. They cited a $5.6 billion charge for coronavirus-related inventory write-offs. They also cited a $4.2 billion revenue reversal because of the return of 7.9 million Paxlovid doses—just from the U.S. government alone. If you didn't think the pharmaceutical industry was "big business", think again. As a result of diminishing sales of its COVID business and these write-offs, Pfizer is looking to make drastic cuts worth $3.5 billion in annual costs by the end of 2024. Pfizer is also seeking to cull and/or move hundreds of its workers from across multiple sites as part of this cost-cutting program. I guess a few bucks spent on some athletes, singers, and influencers is a drop in the bucket to try and right their ship.

Remember, this was never truly about health. This was about money, marketing, and narrative. As I mentioned in an earlier chapter, the "vaccines" were never designed as traditional vaccines. They only respond to the spike protein and not the whole of the virus. If they effectively responded to the 27 proteins inside the virus that make up COVID-19, it would be one and done or a short series and done, much like polio, where the patient has lifetime immunity, or hepatitis B, where you have immunity for 10 years. These shots were never designed like that and the people you put your faith in to make sure the record was clear, people like Anthony Fauci, conveniently left all that information out of their briefings with the press. We saw this immediately and informed our patients that this would be needed yearly, just like the flu shot, but that's not what they heard on television and from the mainstream media. We would sometimes find ourselves arguing with patients about this important fact because the narrative was so strong. The pharmaceutical companies were advertising an effective rate of 95 percent and 77 percent at the time, which led people to gravitate towards the companies touting a 95 percent rate.

Pharmaceutical companies invested significantly in marketing COVID-19 vaccines, but the exact figures can be difficult to pinpoint due to a mix of direct marketing expenditures, government-backed campaigns, and collaborations with public health organizations. Here are some general insights:

1. **Major Campaigns:** In the U.S., pharmaceutical companies like Pfizer and Moderna had extensive marketing efforts, including advertisements on television, digital platforms, and traditional media. Specific figures for Pfizer and Moderna's advertising campaigns in the U.S. were estimated to be in the hundreds of millions of dollars for each company, particularly during the first and second years of the vaccine rollouts (2021-2022).
2. **Government Partnerships:** Many countries, including the U.S., funded public awareness campaigns to promote vaccination. These campaigns sometimes featured pharmaceutical company branding but were often part of broader public health efforts. For instance, the U.S. Department of Health and Human Services (HHS) ran the "We Can Do This" campaign to encourage vaccination, which worked in tandem with pharmaceutical company efforts.

3. **Global Spending Estimates:** Globally, it's estimated that pharmaceutical companies collectively spent billions on marketing COVID-19 vaccines. This figure includes promotional efforts, public relations campaigns, and engagement with healthcare professionals to encourage vaccine adoption. However, a significant portion of the visibility around vaccines also came through earned media and public health campaigns rather than direct advertising spend.

Several celebrities participated in public service announcements, commercials, and campaigns encouraging people to get COVID-19 vaccines. Their involvement was typically part of broader public health efforts, often in partnership with government agencies or nonprofit organizations. Notable celebrities included people like Elton John and Michael Caine. These British icons appeared in a humorous ad together for the UK's National Health Service (NHS) to encourage people to get vaccinated. The lighthearted nature of the commercial was meant to make the message more approachable and relatable. Matthew McConaughey spoke out in various forums, including interviews and social media, to advocate for vaccination, particularly in his home state of Texas. While not specifically in a commercial, his influence as a public figure helped spread the message. Dolly Parton got into the act as well. Although she didn't star in traditional commercials, Parton played a crucial role in promoting COVID-19 vaccines. She helped fund research for the Moderna vaccine and later released a playful video on social media singing a vaccine-themed version of her song "Jolene" while getting vaccinated herself. Stephen Curry, the NBA star, participated in public service announcements encouraging people to get vaccinated. He often used his platform to reach out to younger audiences, discussing the importance of the vaccine for protecting families and communities. Olivia Rodrigo, the singer, collaborated with the White House in 2021 by visiting and participating in public service announcements aimed at younger demographics to encourage vaccination. Jennifer Lopez participated in a campaign in partnership with Global Citizen, a nonprofit organization that worked alongside public health bodies to promote vaccine confidence and equitable distribution worldwide.

I think almost every adult human on the planet knew of or was affected in some way by COVID-19 leading up to the production of the vaccines. COVID-19 wasn't a little-known thing that required the participation of multiple celebrities from across diverse platforms that would appeal to a large demographic. The bottom line is, if people were dying in mass, those who were able to would be lined up for the Covid shots without having to be persuaded by some movie icon or pop singer. Personally, I think the big pharmaceutical companies have too much influence over our elected officials and that conflict of interest is damming. The most likely answer is often the correct answer, and usually the best way to find that answer is to follow the money. Let's look at Pfizer.

- **2022:** Pfizer reported a revenue of approximately **$100.3 billion**.
  - This was a significant increase from previous years, largely driven by COVID-19-related products, especially the Comirnaty (Pfizer-BioNTech COVID-19 vaccine) and Paxlovid, an antiviral COVID-19 treatment.

- **2021:** Pfizer's revenue was about **$81.3 billion**.
  - In 2021, the revenue boost was also primarily attributed to the COVID-19 vaccine, which became one of the top-selling pharmaceuticals in the world during that period.

2. **Net Income:**

- **2022:** Pfizer reported a net income of around **$31.4 billion**.
  - This was a continuation of the strong earnings driven by the widespread sales of their COVID-19-related products.

- **2021:** The net income for 2021 was approximately **$22 billion**.
  - The surge in profits was again related to the global demand for their COVID-19 vaccine.

3. **COVID-19 Product Sales:**

- **Comirnaty (Pfizer-BioNTech COVID-19 vaccine):** In 2022, sales of Comirnaty contributed over **$37 billion** to Pfizer's revenue, down from over **$42 billion** in 2021 as global vaccination rates stabilized and demand varied by region.
- **Paxlovid (COVID-19 antiviral treatment):** The antiviral medication Paxlovid generated around **$18.9 billion** in revenue for Pfizer in 2022.

4. **Research & Development (R&D):**
   - Pfizer has consistently invested in R&D, with

spending in this area being **$11.4 billion** in 2022 and **$10.5 billion** in 2021. A portion of these investments was directed toward the development of COVID-19 treatments and next-generation vaccines.

Overall Financial Impact of the COVID-19 Pandemic

The pandemic significantly boosted Pfizer's financial performance, transforming it into one of the world's highest-grossing pharmaceutical companies during the pandemic years. The demand for vaccines and treatments made COVID-19 products a central part of Pfizer's revenue stream, especially in 2021 and 2022. However, this demand started to decrease by the end of 2022 and into 2023 as vaccination rates stabilized and governments worldwide managed COVID-19 as an endemic issue rather than a pandemic.

Pfizer's contributions to political campaigns are typically made through its **Political Action Committee (PAC)**, known as **Pfizer PAC**. The PAC allows the company to collect voluntary contributions from its employees and use those funds to support political candidates, parties, and committees.

- **Annual Contributions:** The total contributions from Pfizer's PAC vary each election cycle, but they generally range from **$1 million to $2 million** per cycle.
  - For example, in the **2020 election cycle**, Pfizer PAC contributed around **$1.6 million** to federal candidates and committees.
  - Contributions are often split between both major parties in the U.S., with a slight lean depending on the election cycle and the strategic interests of the company.

- In recent cycles, Pfizer's donations have been balanced, with contributions going to both **Democratic** and **Republican** candidates. This approach allows them to maintain relationships across the political spectrum, which is common for large corporations seeking to influence policy.

- **Top Recipients:** Pfizer's contributions often target key members of Congress who are involved in healthcare legislation, pharmaceutical regulation, and business-related policies. These include members of committees like the **Senate Health, Education, Labor, and Pensions (HELP) Committee** and the **House Energy and Commerce Committee**.

Lobbying Expenditures

Pfizer also spends substantial amounts on lobbying efforts, which are separate from campaign contributions but aim to influence legislative and regulatory processes directly:

- **Annual Lobbying Spending:** Pfizer has consistently been among the top pharmaceutical companies in terms of lobbying expenditures.
  - In **2022**, Pfizer spent approximately **$10.5 million** on lobbying activities in the U.S.
  - In **2021**, lobbying expenditures were around **$14.9 million**, a significant increase due to the focus on COVID-19 vaccine-related issues, patent protections, and other regulatory matters.

- **Key Issues for Lobbying: Pfizer's lobbying efforts have focused on a range of issues, including:**
  - **Drug Pricing and Patent Protections:** Advocating for policies that protect intellectual property rights and pricing flexibility for pharmaceuticals.
  - **Regulation of Vaccines and Treatments:** During the COVID-19 pandemic, lobbying efforts centered on vaccine distribution, emergency use authorizations, and securing favorable terms for contracts with the federal government.
  - **Healthcare Policy:** This includes issues related to Medicare and Medicaid, drug reimbursement policies, and broader healthcare reform discussions.

Transparency and Reporting

- Pfizer's contributions and lobbying activities are publicly reported, as required by law. For political contributions, the **Federal Election Commission (FEC)** records donations made by Pfizer's PAC. Lobbying expenditures are reported to the **U.S. Senate** and are accessible through the **Lobbying Disclosure Act Database**.
- These reports offer transparency into how Pfizer uses its resources to support its policy interests and influence political outcomes. As such, the company's involvement in political activities is part of a broader strategy to shape the legislative environment in which it operates.

Pfizer's political spending is a mix of direct contributions through its PAC, generally totaling around **$1-2 million per election cycle**, and more substantial investments in lobbying, with **$10-15 million** spent annually on influencing federal policies.

Moderna was the relatively small player in the COVID-19 vaccine market. Moderna, a biotechnology company, saw significant financial growth during the COVID-19 pandemic, primarily due to the success of its mRNA COVID-19 vaccine, **Spikevax**. The vaccine's sales catapulted the company into a position of high profitability, transforming it from a research-focused biotech company into one of the top players in the pharmaceutical industry. Here's an overview of the financial impact of the pandemic on Moderna:

Key Financial Metrics (2021-2022)

1. **Total Revenue:**
   - **2022:** Moderna reported revenue of approximately **$19.3 billion**.
     - This was primarily driven by sales of the Spikevax COVID-19 vaccine, as demand remained strong, especially for booster doses in many countries.
   - **2021:** Moderna's revenue was around **$18.5 billion**.
     - The revenue in 2021 marked a massive increase compared to pre-pandemic years, as 2021 was the first full year of global vaccine rollout.

2. **Net Income:**
   - **2022:** Moderna reported a net income of about **$8.4 billion**.
   - **2021:** The net income for 2021 was around **$12.2 billion**.

- The year 2021 was particularly profitable for Moderna due to the initial global demand for COVID-19 vaccines, which required widespread primary vaccinations across all age groups.

3. **COVID-19 Vaccine Sales:**
- **Spikevax (Moderna's mRNA COVID-19 Vaccine):**
  - In 2022, sales of Spikevax generated **$18.4 billion** in revenue, a slight increase over 2021 as booster campaigns continued and countries managed additional doses to combat new variants.
  - In 2021, sales of Spikevax accounted for almost all Moderna's **$18.5 billion** in total revenue. This was a dramatic shift for the company, which had never achieved such a high sales volume.

4. **Cash Reserves and Investment:**
- With the profits generated from the vaccine, Moderna significantly increased its cash reserves, reaching over **$18 billion** in cash and cash equivalents by the end of 2022.
- The company has directed a portion of this capital toward research and development (R&D) for other mRNA-based vaccines and therapies, aiming to expand its pipeline beyond COVID-19.

Comparison to Pre-Pandemic Financials

Before the COVID-19 pandemic, Moderna was not yet a revenue-generating company on a significant scale. It was primarily engaged in R&D with no products on the market, generating less than **$100 million** annually from grants and collaborations. The shift to billions in revenue and substantial profitability in 2021 and 2022 marks a dramatic transformation for the company due to its COVID-19 vaccine.

Outlook and Changes in Demand

- As of 2023, demand for COVID-19 vaccines, including those from Moderna, has decreased compared to the peak pandemic years. This is partly due to the widespread availability of initial vaccinations, increased population immunity, and changes in public health approaches to managing COVID-19.
- Moderna's strategy now includes adapting its mRNA platform for new vaccines (such as for flu and RSV) and treatments, aiming to sustain the financial gains it experienced during the pandemic years.

Moderna earned over **$37 billion** in revenue from its COVID-19 vaccine in just two years (2021 and 2022), making substantial profits and transforming its market position. The company's success during the pandemic has provided it with the resources to further invest in its pipeline and continue developing mRNA-based therapeutics.

Overall, I think there may be a bit of cognitive dissonance on the part of the United States Government. When we follow the money they spent, it's no wonder they don't want to admit we had some early data proving that these were unnecessary and ineffective. The amount of taxpayer dollars the United States citizens spent on development, production, and distribution of these shots is staggering!

The U.S. government made substantial investments in COVID-19 vaccines through various contracts and programs to accelerate vaccine development, manufacturing, and distribution. Here is an overview of the key expenditures related to COVID-19 vaccines:

1. Operation Warp Speed (OWS)

- **Initial Investment:** The U.S. government launched Operation Warp Speed (OWS) in May 2020 to accelerate the development, production, and distribution of COVID-19 vaccines. It involved a combination of federal agencies, including the Department of Health and Human Services (HHS), the Department of Defense (DOD), and private pharmaceutical companies.
- **Total Budget:** The total budget for OWS was about **$18 billion**, which covered vaccine research, development, manufacturing, and distribution efforts for multiple companies.
- **Vaccine Purchases:** OWS provided upfront funding to vaccine manufacturers like Pfizer-BioNTech, Moderna, and Johnson & Johnson, reducing their financial risk and expediting vaccine availability for the American public.

2. Contracts with Vaccine Manufacturers

The U.S. government signed contracts worth tens of billions of dollars to purchase COVID-19 vaccines. Here's a breakdown of some of the key contracts:

- **Pfizer-BioNTech:**
  - The U.S. government made multiple agreements with Pfizer-BioNTech for vaccine doses, with contracts totaling approximately **$30 billion** by 2023. This covered the purchase of doses for initial vaccination, booster shots, and updated vaccines for new variants.
  - Each dose was initially purchased for about **$19.50** but later increased to between **$24 to $30** per dose for subsequent contracts.

- **Moderna:**
  - Moderna received funding for development and purchase agreements totaling around **$10-15 billion** for doses supplied to the U.S. government.
  - Moderna's initial contracts priced doses around **$15-16** each, with costs for booster doses increasing over time.

- **Johnson & Johnson (Janssen):**
  - The U.S. government allocated around **$1-2 billion** for doses of the Johnson & Johnson vaccine, which was later limited in use due to rare blood clot risks.
  - The contract covered up to **100 million doses**, but fewer were ultimately used compared to mRNA vaccines from Pfizer-BioNTech and Moderna.

- **Novavax and Other Vaccine Manufacturers:**
  - Contracts with other companies, including Novavax, also contributed to the government's total expenditures on vaccines. However, these vaccines played a more minor role compared to Pfizer and Moderna.

3. Additional Costs for Distribution and Administration

- **Distribution and Logistics:** Beyond the purchase of vaccines, significant funds were allocated to the logistics of vaccine distribution, including the supply chain, cold storage, and delivery to vaccination sites. This also covered partnerships with companies like McKesson for distribution and logistics.
- **Administration Costs:** The U.S. government funded efforts to administer the vaccines, including supporting state and local health departments, vaccine clinics, pharmacies, and mobile vaccination units. These efforts included paying for the administration fees for shots, even when the vaccines themselves were provided at no cost to the recipients.

4. Total Estimated Expenditure on Vaccines

- **Total Direct Spending:** Estimates for the total U.S. spending on COVID-19 vaccines, including purchase contracts, logistics, and administration, are around **$40-50 billion** through the end of 2022.
- This includes initial purchases under Operation Warp Speed as well as subsequent purchases of booster doses and variant-specific vaccines.

5. Support for Global Vaccination Efforts

- In addition to domestic spending, the U.S. government also contributed to global vaccination efforts through initiatives like **COVAX** (COVID-19 Vaccines Global Access). The U.S. pledged **$4 billion** to support COVAX and donated surplus doses to other countries to help improve global vaccine access.

Summary of U.S. Spending on COVID-19 Vaccines

The U.S. government's investment in COVID-19 vaccines was substantial, with around **$40-50 billion** directed toward domestic vaccine development, purchase, and distribution efforts, and an additional **$4 billion** to support global vaccination. This investment is hard to walk away from considering it was touted as the only way to combat the pandemic and the investment was supported by almost every single member of Congress.

It may now seem like any additional expenditure is just a cover because nobody wants to admit that this was a giant waste of time and money. I think the biggest dupe of them all is the fact that the government changed the definition of the word "vaccine" in this exercise, making people feel like they were going to get inoculated during this process. When the vaccine manufacturers reported a 95 or 77 percent efficacy rate, the public assumed that these shots worked according to what they thought was a traditional definition of the word vaccine. The public didn't need to have expertise in this field, but they should have let those of us who did have expertise explain the facts to them without censorship.

In the fog of war, the public was duped, governments were duped, and the pharmaceutical companies made out like bandits. All the celebrities who participated have enough plausible deniability to keep most of their credibility intact because the mainstream narrative supported their effort. However, the voices of the people who have had vaccine injuries fall on deaf ears because most who were duped in this process are too prideful to come out and admit it. The momentum will eventually shift as new studies prove what most are thinking and the data is compiled to show cause and correlation, but by then, it will be too late for most except the large pharmaceutical companies. They are laughing all the way to the bank.

12

WHAT THE NURSES ARE SAYING

You May Want to Pay Attention!

The data alone paints a bleak picture, but it's not the entire story. While most of the metrics never make it into the VAERS system, the stories that the nurses tell can be even more unsettling. There is a stark difference between nursing practices from the time before Covid and now, specifically in regard to the vaccine rollouts. This chapter explores where we are today in comparison to before the Covid pandemic. A lot has changed in medicine, and not for the better.

I've had the opportunity to speak to nurses and practitioners all over the country about the changes they have seen and continue to see. Most of them want to remain anonymous for fear of reprisals. In addition to some of the physical changes they have seen in patients, most report a complete change in attitude and mental state among the staff. What's important to note is that while I was interested in some of the anomalies associated with the Covid vaccines, a lot of the nurses and practitioners point to the totality of the circumstances with the entirety of the post-Covid era. I think there is a distinct tie in between the two, and you may be surprised at what you hear.

Mental and Physical Exhaustion

When Covid first reared its head, a lot of primary care offices shut their doors for fear that these practitioners would bring Covid home to their own families. This overwhelmed the hospital systems. Emergency rooms began to overflow with non-emergency cases, which put a giant strain on the number of hospital staff, particularly the nurses, who were now seeing a much higher volume of patients. Before Covid, the norm for a nurse-to-patient ratio was one nurse to every four patients and ranged up to one nurse to six patients. That has since increased and continues to get higher. At the time of writing, four years after the pandemic began, that ratio is anywhere from one to six to about one to ten in some cases. The medical staff tells me that any more than six patients per nurse on a shift is unsafe.

Due to the COVID-19 mandates, an abundance of nurses who were slated for retirement within the next 10 years, decided to call it quits. Some of these nurses did their best to seek out exemptions from the vaccine mandates but were largely unsuccessful. In fact, hospital staffing mandates were often tied to Federal payments. Hospital systems were told that if they did not get at least an 80 percent participation rate from their staff they would lose their payments from Medicare. Medicare is usually the system's largest payer.

Additionally, approximately 100,000 nurses left the workforce in the United States due to the heightened stress, burnout, and challenging working conditions. The pandemic significantly worsened existing issues in the nursing profession, including unsafe staffing levels, emotional exhaustion, and increased workloads. Projections indicate that nearly 900,000 nurses could leave the profession by 2027, posing serious challenges to healthcare systems nationwide if further support and retention efforts are not implemented.

The pandemic acted as a catalyst for many nurses to exit the field, highlighting the need for systemic reforms to reduce burnout and improve workplace environments. These developments reflect broader concerns about workforce shortages, which continue to strain healthcare facilities and limit patient care capacity. As one nurse put it, "When you come into an emergency room, instead of complaining to the staff that the wait is so long, look around you. Do you see anybody hemorrhaging? Are you witnessing a woman giving birth in a chair? NO, you're not! Emergency rooms have turned into modern day primary care. You could be sitting there with severe abdominal pain, but you may look just like the guy sitting next to you that ran out of his blood pressure medication. Emergency rooms don't turn people away, and if you truly have an emergency, there may not be the room nor the staffing to tend to your needs as fast as you may have been used to."

Disbelief in diagnosis

I've pointed out in my writings that it was tough for me to fight the battle of the narrative. The fact that you could get or give Covid once a patient had been "vaccinated" was something we knew early on. However, I had been challenged by several patients who were in disbelief about their positive results. The same went for masks in the beginning. I would often call a patient to tell them they were positive only to be met with the words, "I don't understand how I have it, I've been wearing a mask the whole time." As frustrating as this was for me, the hospital staff had to deal with it one on one and sometimes with the entirety of the patients' family chiming in. One female nurse said, "Patients were told that receiving the vaccine was like a coat of armor against Covid. When vaccinated patients came in and tested positive for Covid, we were called liars! We had a patient who was maxed out on nasal cannula oxygen and had to call respiratory for an Opti Flo (high flow nasal oxygen therapy), and we were asked by his wife, who was panicking, why this was happening. We made her aware that her husband was in fact positive for Covid. She wanted the Opti Flo cancelled and for him to be given time to calm down. She had their vaccine cards in her hand and was yelling that she was being lied to because there was NO WAY he had Covid."

When a patient is hypoxic, you must act quickly to keep their oxygen level up. There is simply no time for negotiations, but the confusion surrounding the Covid vaccines complicated the normal workflow of the medical staff. She continued, "Us nurses once led the nation in ratings for honesty and ethics for 20 straight years. We lost that once Covid hit. When you lose trust from your patients, it makes your job very difficult."

Lack of Trust

Losing the trust of your patients because you or your team did something wrong may be understandable, but losing the trust of your patients because the government and media couldn't get the narrative right was even more frustrating. One female nurse said, "I had a hospice patient who had been tested for Covid upon entry. Her daughter looked me right in the eye and said, 'I hope you go on a glamorous vacation with your Covid bonus, although we know my mom is passing from a brain bleed." As a nurse, here you are helping someone cross over pain-free, and the family members are convinced that we were receiving bonuses for Covid deaths. The patient wasn't a Covid death, it was a brain bleed, but because the protocol was to test everyone at the time for Covid, when she tested positive, even though it was secondary to the brain bleed, the family members acted like we just got handed a lottery ticket."

When the vaccines came out, there was so much misinformation floating around that most people thought they would be completely inoculated against COVID-19. As I've explained, the truth was and is that they work like a flu shot, giving you limited resistance against a specific spike protein. The lack of communication and the dishonest narrative that the CDC was disseminating was making it very hard for the practitioners to relay the reality of what we saw firsthand. It was like we were fighting against the tide and the current all at the same time—and drowning in the process.

While most of the population couldn't wait to rush out and get these shots as soon as they became available, there was another segment of the population that was skeptical of them and thought we were all part of the conspiracy. Another nurse said, "During med pass, I was going over all scheduled medications with a patient for accuracy. Heparin is a blood thinner that is given every eight hours subcutaneously while patients are on bed rest to prevent clots. The patient agreed to get her Heparin shot, so I drew it up, and when I walked to the side of her bed, she kicked me right in the stomach because she said I was giving her a Covid vaccine without her consent. I got the Heparin bottle and showed her it. She then told me to get out and said, "I know what you people are about!"

We heard the same sort of things while testing. People would accuse us of having microchips in swabs or that the swabs were contaminated. The dichotomy of people during this time was incredible. In my opinion, it seemed to get worse after the vaccine rollouts. It pitted citizen against citizen, the vaccinated against the unvaccinated. For most of the people who didn't want the vaccine, it just came down to a personal choice or an educated one. The ones who rushed out and got them were just relying on blind luck, and more importantly, were acting out of fear. Fear can drive a narrative, even with no scientific evidence to back up the claims. Now those fears are causing more long-term health issues.

People putting health concerns at bay

Even after the "vaccine" rollout, the country didn't just magically go back to normal. There were many delays in care for people who most desperately needed it. Let's take diabetics for instance. Many diabetic patients develop non-healing wounds that require consistent medical attention. One nurse spoke of such cases by saying, "We're seeing just as many amputations in diabetics, if not more, as we did back in the 1980s. When medications and treatments are readily available, amputations should be very infrequent. Even after the vaccines came out, patients still had to show a negative Covid swab on top of a vaccine card to get into a wound care facility. Wound care facilities limited their hours for exposure risk, and by the time they reopened fully, these patients had already been admitted to the hospital and needed a higher level of care."

Take, for instance, an older patient with a hip fracture who needed rehabilitation. The Covid vaccine mandates didn't do much to help with their care either. The same nurse stated, "Patients that were cleared for rehab needed three consecutive negative Covid tests before being accepted into a facility." It's now clear to see that the pandemic and complications surrounding the vaccine mandates and rollouts caused widespread issues that contributed to the downfall of many patients' healthcare. The frightening stories are coming out now that the masses have received these experimental shots.

Mysterious illnesses

Everyone seems to have a Covid story about a person they know, or even themselves, that seems a little out of the ordinary. I told a story in *Fauci's Fiction* about a patient who received the Pfizer shots and almost immediately started to get joint inflammation. Her hands swelled up to where she couldn't get her engagement ring off. The second shot caused even more problems almost immediately after receiving her dose.

However, the stories coming out of the hospitals nationwide are incredible. One nurse told me, "I had a 28-year-old male admitted for dehydration, vomiting, nausea and diarrhea. He had been exhibiting these symptoms for the last 72 hours. All his basic labs and blood cultures were normal. He couldn't keep any food down, so the doctors on staff sent the patient down for a CT scan. They thought they might see pancreatitis and start a plan of care from there, but he had a tumor the size of a grapefruit woven throughout his intestine. The tumor was inoperable at this phase of growth, and the patient decided to go with hospice care to make him comfortable. So this poor guy came in thinking he had a virus, and once admitted, he never left the hospital ever again." Of course, I had to ask how many shots this patient had received. She answered, "Four shots, which if you understood why, kills me. This patient worked for a landscaping company, OUTSIDE, and his landscaping company was worried about losing their clients if their staff were unvaccinated."

    The recurrence of cancers we are hearing about is one of the things that sticks out most in my mind. I mentioned my dear friend Marilyn earlier. Her scans were all clear and then, all of a sudden, out of nowhere, she developed a giant tumor in her esophagus which led to her death. One nurse told me, "A woman was diagnosed with stage two breast cancer in 2010. She had the tumor removed and went through treatment with a clean bill of health. Four to six months after receiving her Covid shots, she discovered a lump in her right breast while showering. Due to her history, she panicked. She went to her doctor and scheduled a biopsy due to her past medical history and found out she was in stage four cancer after over ten years of being clean. They immediately scheduled her for a double mastectomy and chemotherapy. She was in her mid-thirties and a stay-at-home mom with three kids who had gotten vaccinated so she could take her kids to Disney."

Complications for even something like asthma seems to be getting worse. One nurse stated, "We've had people who were diagnosed with asthma and given a rescue inhaler, but they would never even use them before they expire. Now we see these asthmatics coming in with attacks, but if you look at their medication list, they are on four or five inhalers. Since the vaccines came out, their asthma can't be controlled.

The truly disturbing thing is what everyone tells me about the age range of these patients. When I spoke to Richard Hirschman, he pointed out that he was embalming more young people than ever, and he had noticed a very stark difference in the age groups and the number of young people he was seeing now compared to previously in his 20-year career. I am hearing the same exact story from the nurses who care for these patients first.

One nurse said, "We see everything from irregular heart rhythms to younger and younger patients going to the Cath lab to receive a stent. We see heart attacks in younger and younger patients. Cardiology is always onboarded for older patients, but seeing it for our younger population will never sit well with me. Pre-Covid, the average patient going to the Cath lab was probably in their mid-40s, and even that was considered young. Now there are kids in their 20s going to the Cath lab daily. We had an 18-year-old high school football player whose father thought he was complaining of a pulled muscle in his leg. When he came to the hospital, he could barely bear any weight on his left leg. An ultrasound was done and was positive for micro clots. The patient was placed on a Heparin drip and was admitted for a week, and now needs to be placed on a daily blood thinner to prevent any future clotting.

Of course, he needed his shots because his school mandated them to play sports."

The same nurse was upfront about her observations over the last few years. She said, "Imagine being forced to get a shot to keep your job and then caring for patients that are receiving vaccine injuries, in all ages, and all sexes. It kind of fucks with you a little bit. These shots didn't discriminate. At first, you thought it was yourself being hyper-sensitive, but once you started hearing the doctors talking about it, it started to become a reality. The doctors were asking more questions like, "What vaccine did you get? How long ago did you get it? Was your temperature checked before you received it?" Then you realize at that point, this is the new norm, and you just wonder what's next."

There are still people who just don't get it. They are blinded by the government and media's initial narrative and think everyone else around them must be lying or trying to spin what the reality is. One nurse told me about a middle-aged woman who just didn't want to listen to medical advice. She said, "This woman was in the hospital being treated for a DVT (deep vein thrombosis, or clot) and wanted to receive the Covid booster before she left. The patient was told that the vaccine was contra-indicated at this time. The patient stated that Covid was a concern of hers and she wanted her booster. She said that if we wouldn't give it, she would stop at her local pharmacy to get it on her way home." Ironically, this patient was most likely hospitalized because of getting these shots in the first place. The amount of blot clots we've seen since the "vaccine" rollouts has been staggering. This is probably why you've heard them being called the "clot shots".

As I mentioned earlier, the belief in these "vaccines" was also an issue for hospital staff. We knew you could get Covid and transmit Covid after a person received their shots. It didn't help that President Biden was the most predominant person to deny this publicly, and yes, the video is out there, but most of them have been scrubbed from YouTube. One nurse told me, "We had a Covid-positive patient requiring oxygen due to hypoxia. While walking out of the patient's room and removing my PPE, his wife was walking up to visit. She asked why I was dressed like that while looking me up and down. I told her it was hospital protocol for all Covid-positive patients. She replied with, "Didn't anyone tell you he was vaccinated?" Then she laughed and said what I was doing was completely unnecessary. She attempted to enter his room without even wearing an N-95 mask, but I told her that this was not allowed. With that, she told me that she too was vaccinated and closed the door on me." She continued, "It's hard to believe that people listened so intently to Dr. Fauci and President Biden over their own personal medical staff who were caring for them at the bedside. I wanted to say, "If I'm a liar, then how do you even feel safe with me taking care of your family member?"

It's ironic that people only wanted to pay attention to certain doctors. There were very good doctors out there who had a lot more experience with Covid and these shots. Those doctors and nurses were saying very different things than what was on the mainstream news. The mainstream media was repeating the CDC narrative, and the doctors who went along with that narrative all got it wrong! It was the outliers who had it right, and more importantly, the people who had the vast amount of experience with Covid patients The ones who were guessing were incorrect and led a lot of sheep to their slaughter. I always say, when someone tells you something, you should ask what they are basing their premise on. Most of the people screaming about Covid have no basis for their arguments, and now a lot of unwilling followers continue to carry their water.

One nurse said, "Nobody wanted to be educated on what was being seen. They had all their faith in that shot. With the flu shot, people know that they still have the possibility of getting the flu, but with this, they were convinced that there was absolutely no way that they would ever be Covid-positive. There were good sales tactics on that."

The number of rare cancers that we've been seeing is something I would never be able to emphasize without writing a 500-page book, the stories are abundant. The number of rare cancers in younger patients is astonishing. The things the nurses are seeing today are vastly different from the norms they were used to before Covid, and more importantly, before the shots were rolled out. I hear countless stories that include lines such as "I've never seen anything like this before" from just about every medical staffer I talk to. The nurses, though, see so many patients through their shifts, and they eventually start to talk to each other about the amount of craziness that they are witnessing.

One nurse told me the story of a patient in his teens. The patient was diagnosed with Thymoma. This is a very slow-growing cancerous tumor in the Thymus. The thymus is a small gland in the upper chest, about two inches long at birth, but shrinks as you age through a process called involution. At puberty, the thymus reaches its largest weight at about one ounce. By age 60, the Thymus weighs about half that. Its location is in the upper front of the chest behind the sternum and extends upwards towards the neck. The thymus's size and function decrease with age, which can lead to an increased risk of disease. The nurse said, "Thymomas are very rare and usually seen in patients older than 70. This kid was telling the team that he felt something when he swallowed in his chest wall. When they did the scans, it looked like his thymus was the size of an apple or baseball. These tumors are very slow-growing, which is why they usually get discovered when someone is in their 70s. Here's a kid at 16 with this large, rare tumor that is growing at a rapid rate. The doctors stated that they had never seen anything like that before."

When you listen to the stories and you talk to the staff who've done this before and after the "vaccine" rollouts, you hear some interesting yet scary tales. The same nurse summed up the totality of what she'd been seeing by saying, "When I think about the time and effort I put into educating people on medications, it amazes me that people would just walk into a pharmacy to get a vaccine that's brand new. I think the vaccine gave people a false sense of security. These shots never protected people the way they thought they were going to. It weakened their systems, just like Covid does! So, people were afraid of Covid, yet they rolled up their sleeves without asking any questions. I feel like, when you used to talk, people would listen. Now, I feel like people gravitate towards certain words and have a lot of distrust in the medical community. I feel like the medical community is personally being blamed. I feel like they are grouping the government and medicine into one because they are looking for someone to blame. In every specialty, we see heightened cases. Heightened meaning, more cancer, more psychological issues, more arrhythmias, more anemia, everything is more! It's probably safe to say we are seeing triple the number of cases than we were seeing before the entirety of the pandemic. Patients used to be seen in the emergency room and then leave the same day. Now they are in the hospital for three to four days, and it's taking longer to figure out a proper plan of care. We used to be able to see a patient, pinpoint the issue, develop a plan of care, treat them, and send them on their way. For example, it's no longer basic UTI's we're seeing. Now the UTI's stem from kidney problems, but the patient is hypertensive, so that is causing kidney problems. It's now a maze of hard stops on something that used to be very basic to treat. Instead of having a primary care physician treat a UTI, you now have a nephrologist and a cardiologist to take care of a basic condition. Medicine has become more complex."

The stories are endless, and I suspect they will continue for a long time to come. The anomalies seemed to have calmed slightly as most people have woken up to realize they don't need these things in their bodies to stay safe, but there most certainly is a correlation between the shots being rolled out and the massive amount of data being collected on vaccine injuries. It's not a narrative, it's a reality. For the naysayers, argue with the data, argue with the evidence. I'll never understand why you would run out and get the latest booster that doesn't work as advertised and has caused more harm than the actual disease. You can admit you were wrong; it may make you more likeable...

13

MY BUDDY PHIL

If you read my first book, *Fauci's Fiction*, you would know the story of my dear friends Phillip and Marilyn Perricone. In an earlier chapter, I wrote about Marilyn's death, but books take a long time to write, and tragically, her husband and my dear friend passed just a few months after his wife did. They both passed in the same year, and of course, there is a relationship with Covid to discuss. It was only a few weeks before writing this chapter that I told Phil I had written about Marilyn in this book. I said, "Phil, you know how much we loved Marilyn, and since you were both a focus in my first book about the Pandemic, it's only fitting that I mention Marilyn and immortalize her in this new book." He smiled and said, "Good, I'm glad," and never even once pondered what I may reveal. The questionable circumstances regarding Marilyn's cancer coming back so quickly and with the virulence it did left us all wondering if it was caused by all the Covid shots she had received. Phil, on the other hand, was a very different story.

My world has been rocked by some close personal deaths over the last 18 months. First, my father passed away quickly and without warning. My first book is dedicated to him, and I am certain that the Covid shots were a contributing factor in his death. Then we were rocked by Marilyn's cancer returning after receiving clean scans just six months prior. A few months later, my mother passed away suddenly, and then just another few short months later we lost Phil. The one thing they all had in common was that they had all received multiple Covid shots and boosters. I lost both my parents and a couple that I regarded as some of my closest friends, although my wife says they were just like another set of parents. In fact, we spent just about every holiday with Phil and Marilyn. Christmas dinners, Thanksgiving, the 4th of July... You name it, we were either at their house down the street, at an event, or even at a Country Club if everyone was too busy to cook that year. Phil would just make reservations, and without fail, we were all together. Life won't quite be the same in our household ever again.

Just two weeks ago, Phil was scheduled to fly into New Jersey and stay at our house. This was common after he had sold his home in New Jersey and moved to Florida full-time. When Phil came to town, he would try to make the rounds and see everyone, but he would usually stay with us in our guest room. He texted me the morning he was supposed to arrive and said, "Needed to cancel the trip. Think I have Covid or bad flu. Going to doc this morning." My response was, "Sorry to hear that, we were looking forward to seeing you." He replied, "Shit happens!" We went on with our day. About an hour later, Phil reached out to my wife by text, saying, "Went to the doc, have Covid." As Kelly was reading this to me, I immediately started boiling. I couldn't reach for my phone quickly enough. Phil had read my book, *Fauci's Fiction,* TWICE, and we had discussed it ad nausea over the last four years, so I was ready for a battle.

Phil wasn't in the best of health. He had uncontrolled diabetes, numerous other health concerns, and smoked like a chimney. I had always said, if you are in the pool of the population that is susceptible to dying in the next five years, a cold can bring you down, the flu can bring you down, Covid can bring you down... However, we weren't sure that Phil even had Covid. You see, as I've talked about in previous chapters, you CANNOT diagnose Covid on a rapid antigen test. A rapid antigen test can come back as positive for any Coronavirus we test for—there are seven on our respiratory panel. You also need a huge amount of viral load to trigger a rapid antigen test. See the chapter in *Fauci's Fiction* titled "How Testing Actually Works, There's More to it than You Think."

I immediately called Phil and said, "What do you mean you have Covid? You obviously had a rapid test since it came back so quickly, did they test you for anything else?" He told me they had also tested him for the flu. I said, "Phil, there are 31 things on a respiratory pathogen panel, so what about the other 29?" The fact is, he may have had Covid, but he was symptomatic, so they didn't test him for any co-infections he most likely had. In all our data in testing over 19,000 patients, the sickest of the sick ALWAYS had a co-infection. Phil said, "I know, I know, I told them no to the Paxlovid but what else could you have done, Mike?" I said, "If you were here, I would have done an RPP and found out EXACTLY what you have so we could prescribe an antibiotic for any bacterial infection you may also have, in addition, if you are that symptomatic, there are other things we can do to mitigate the inflammation."

He could hear the frustration in my voice because he'd heard me say, on more than one occasion, that the entire medical community hasn't learned a thing about what we just went through. He walked into an urgent care which has no follow up and cannot bill for a follow-up appointment, so why would they bother to do anything other than a rapid covid and flu test? It's sheer stupidity in the totality of the circumstances, and Phil was at that age and in that pool of the population that we discussed. If nothing else, and because of his underlying conditions, they should have given him a chest x-ray and checked if there were any abnormalities heard in his lung sounds. I was annoyed because we had done this thousands of times, and there he was, over 1000 miles away with some doc in a box trying to rush him in and out without having a history on him. There wasn't much I could do from our position, but we confidently figured he would be okay.

We had a charity event with Phil on the calendar that week, and he asked us to keep our obligation in his absence as he had purchased a table for all of us to attend. We obliged, and a few days later, we showed up at the event. His son Rob was there, along with some of his former neighbors and friends. I had spoken to him two days earlier, and he told me that he was feeling slightly better. His friend Susan came up to me at the event to tell me that she had spoken to him earlier that day and he was almost back to normal. I remember everyone coming up to me to tell me that Phil had Covid, and my response was, "No, Phil thinks he had Covid, but we do not have a confirmatory test, so we really don't know what Phil has." In fact, when you do this for a living and write an entire book about a pandemic that EVERYONE wanted answers to back in 2020 but doesn't seem to care about anymore, it's severely frustrating. When I was the first in my state to start conducting testing back in 2020, I felt like I was alone on an island. Just four short years later, I felt the same way. I felt like NOBODY HAS LEARNED A DAM THING!

Our mutual friend Peter had intended to head down to Phil's house in Florida the following week. My wife and I had to travel there as well but would be about an hour away filming our shows, so it wasn't plausible in our schedules to visit Phil. I was confident that Pete would take charge of things and make sure Phil was on the mend. When we landed in Florida a few days later, I called Phil to check on him but got no answer. I was confident that Pete was in town and maybe the two of them were catching up, so I didn't think too much about it. We spent a few days filming for the show we are doing on Rumble and traveled back to New Jersey. On Monday, I woke up to do my live show and almost immediately after I was clear, my phone rang—it was Peter. Pete and I talk all the time, and I figured he was catching up to ask how our trip went and how much I missed out on not being able to go see them. I could immediately tell that something was up by Peter's voice, and that's when he told me that Phil was gone. Pete had never made the trip because Phil told him not to come, that he wasn't feeling 100 percent. Pete and Phil's son Rob only found out after the authorities made a wellness visit because they were unable to contact Phil.

This is when the what-ifs and should-I-haves started to play in my mind... If only I had known that he had a little more going on, maybe we could have rescheduled and gone down to take care of him. Even though Phil was feeling better from what we think was a viral infection, he had a nasty cough. Those coughs can linger when someone has co-morbidities like Phil, hell, they lingered with me on more than one occasion after getting ill. Unbeknownst to me, Phil had esophageal varices. These are abnormal veins that run from the tube running from the throat to the stomach. They usually develop when blood flow to the liver is blocked. There are usually no symptoms unless the veins bleed, but in previous instances with Phil, they had. He'd had some coughing spats where he started to cough up blood and had to be seen for advanced medical care. His illness probably inflamed this condition, and his coughing may have caused these varices to burst. When he was found in bed, he was covered in blood from coughing these up, and his phone was on the other side of the house in the kitchen. He may have gone to bed thinking nothing was wrong and woke up in a coughing fit that caused his untimely passing. We will never truly know, and as this death wasn't suspicious due to his age and because it was from natural causes, this case was not one for the medical examiner. No autopsy was performed, and his death will be recorded as unremarkable. Additionally, there was no examination of his wife Marilyn or my mother. My father was the only one out of the four who had an autopsy performed, and in his case, there is a strong likelihood the vaccines were a contributing factor in his death. In Phil's case, anything is plausible, but I am more concerned about the lack of efficacy in treatment that contributed to his death.

The respective ages of these four deaths that surrounded me over the last 18 months were 75, 76, 77, and 78. In my mind, way too young, given all the advancements in healthcare we have currently. We will never know if the shots contributed to some of their deaths because there is no smoking gun, but it's always a suspicion in the back of my mind, especially after everything I've seen throughout my own research and with our patient population. Again, I never recommended the Covid "vaccine" for two reasons, not because I thought it would have a detrimental effect on the recipient, but because it wasn't needed, and it didn't work. Those two reasons are overwhelmingly powerful reasons to not put an experimental drug into the masses with no long-term testing. Why would I give you something experimental that I already knew, from our patient population, DIDN'T WORK? Why would I recommend something experimental for you for something that EVERY single one of my patients recovered from? To push the mainstream narrative was simply illogical!

It was sad to watch this entire group over the last four years, fearful of a virus they couldn't see, but something I knew an abundance about. I watched them change their whole lives and rush out to get the "shots" because they wanted the chance to live. Sadly, it wouldn't be long before they didn't have that chance anymore. It's hard knowing more than those around you and fighting to relay that knowledge when the whole of the mainstream media and government is against you. My friend Phil learned most of what I knew in real time as we spoke often, and I wasn't shy about trying to help those who were confused about what they saw on that CNN death count they kept running up the ratings with. Even after I published a book about Covid, it's still hard to break through the narrative that was drilled into everyone's head. What's even worse is that, much of the time, I must explain my work differently to different people depending on what they think or if they have gone down a specific rabbit hole. If that challenge wasn't daunting enough, the government is still pushing much of the same narrative on people in the age group that are most susceptible to the end of life.

Phil would always look at me with a sense of bewilderment when I would talk about COVID-19, as if I was reaching to cherry-pick a narrative just to go against the grain. What he didn't realize, in all our years of friendship, was that I care more about my credibility than anything. I'm in the public eye, I have lifelong relationships that I value deeply. My credibility means the world to me, and I wouldn't say or stake my reputation on something unless I had ALL the facts because I wouldn't want it to come back to bight me in the ass later. Can you imagine how unbelievably frustrating it is when you are trying to protect your parents and friends from danger you can clearly see but they cannot? While they are looking at you like you have three heads, you are thinking in your mind, "I wouldn't be saying this out loud if I didn't have all the facts to back it up!" By the way, "What do you do for a living?"

It took Phil a while and a lot of doing for himself to realize that my constant dissertations were based on merit. Phil and Marilyn had gotten the shots, and they still caught Covid, despite the narrative that you "couldn't get it nor give it". Yes, that was said and yes, that clip has become much harder to find on the internet. The bottom line is people believed it... We knew then that the "vaccines" being developed only targeted the spike protein, therefore anyone could catch and transmit COVID-19 after getting "vaccinated". We knew then from the daily calls to all our patients that people were still catching COVID-19 in abundance even after being "fully vaccinated". We knew then that people were getting just as sick who had been "fully vaccinated", and we knew in real time that the mortality rate stayed the same from the time before the shots rolled out until after—and that remains true today.

Phil was a smart guy, a business guy in the marine electronics industry for many years. He was hugely successful and spent a lot of his time in retirement giving back, especially to the local hospital system, where he proudly sat on the board. When I say I was alone on an island, I can't emphasize that enough. It was little ol' me against the world, but the world that was touting all this nonsense to Phil didn't have any real-time patient data. I couldn't figure out why someone like my buddy Phil would doubt the things I was telling him from my own, very large data set. It wasn't like we had five patients and just told him my "hunch" about what we thought. I was telling him about my observations from thousands and thousands of real patients that we had actual follow-up conversations with daily.

After the dust settled on Covid and Marilyn's cancer returned, none of the bickering about Covid seemed to matter anymore. Life is precious and very short. When Marilyn put two and two together in our last conversation, I felt bad, the goal wasn't to "be right". The goal was to save my friends and protect them from what I saw others getting sick from. If I said it once, I said it a thousand times to my dad, my mother, and Phil and Marilyn, "You don't want those shots, you don't need those shots, you're going to get Covid anyway, and you'll be fine, just like the other 19,000 patients I've had." I told them about my hypothesis with my immunologist about getting multiple cytokine reactions from multiple shots and theoretically being worse off once you catch Covid because your body has had multiple, unnecessary inflammatory responses. I spoke to them about my patient data, anecdotal stories, and how ridiculous the narrative seemed, but the bottom line is, the narrative makers were just louder than me. Right around the time Marilyn passed away, Phil said publicly that I was the smartest guy he knew. He said he still had the post-it notes I wrote on to predict the spread of Covid back in March 2020 and couldn't understand how I was able to foresee all that so very early. He told me how proud my father would have been for the work that I was doing, if only my father knew. That meant more to me than anything, as Phil absolutely loved my dad and was one of the last connections I had to my father in this world.

    I watched this entire group of family and friends set aside their normal lives to "stay home to stay safe", to "mask up for our children", and to "get vaccinated to stop the spread". In the meantime, they didn't travel much, they didn't go out. They washed their groceries, limited time with friends and family, avoided funerals for loved ones, avoided public spaces, and most of all, just stopped LIVING! It was a tough time to watch your friends do this when my family and I were doing EVERYTHING in our power to make sure we were enjoying life to its fullest. We knew this thing wasn't going to destroy us, so once we knew the real dangers, we forged on to make sure we enjoyed life while everyone else was locked away or dealing with the anxiety of Fauci's fiction.

Even if the vaccine didn't contribute to Phil's passing, the entire exercise limited some of his life in his final years, and that's not acceptable. In Marilyn's case, I truly believe that she wouldn't have developed the cancer at such a rapid rate if she hadn't run out for those shots. That's what she was trying to tell me during our last conversation... Could have, would have, well, who knows? If the choice were different, would it have been a different outcome? I think anyone laying sick and faced with death at any moment would question the choices they made and think back to those many conversations that we had. Marilyn's death was also something that was weighing on Phil and didn't contribute to his overall health. The entirety of the last four years seemed to be a chain reaction that all started in Wuhan, China and exploded around the world just to end with a thud. What's funny is, the cases are still out there, Covid hasn't gone away. The mortality rate is exactly what I predicted it to be back in March 2020, but all the hysteria, the mask wearing, the grocery washing, and the disruption to life has disappeared. What's worse is, so have my family and friends. What we wouldn't all do to get that time back and have more time moving forward. When someone asks me what my most valuable asset is, I tell them, "It's my time." I guess that's a perspective on life, but I'm also quite sure my buddy Phil would have the same answer.

14

TAKEAWAYS

WHEN I WOKE UP THIS MORNING, I saw another headline that read, "Pfizer Covid booster jab leaves fit man, 54, in chronic pain." The article continued, the man "was fit and regularly ran 10km at a time before he took the Pfizer Covid booster." A few years after the rollout of the Covid shots, stories like this have become common place. I'm not sure if anybody is paying attention and I think there is a certain segment of the population that just ignores them. The one thing I would have done differently in *Fauci's Fiction* would be to wrap up everything in a nice little bow. The reception of the book was great, but too many of my readers didn't put all the pieces of the puzzle together. At least, not well enough for me to say I had done my job. This pandemic affected everyone in the world in some way. Most people are still very confused about what exactly happened, and the story is far from written. I wanted to make sure that in this book, which will be my last on the subject, I put everything I possibly could into perspective for you and give you my thoughts on some of the more important aspects of the vaccines and the COVID-19 pandemic itself.

The Most Important Thing we Learned

For three years, we went through one of the largest unplanned case studies in the history of respiratory pathogens. My team and I tested over 19,000 patients and conducted over 44,000 tests, which was technically unnecessary, but it allowed us to put all respiratory pathogens into perspective—and we will, most likely, never have that opportunity again. We learned that just about everyone is walking around with some kind of infection during some portion of their life, and people most likely never know it! People get staff infections like Staph Aureus all the time and would never know. They usually clear up on their own, and the same goes for a host of other pathogens. Look around next time you are in a public place. At least 10 percent of the people around you are most likely fighting off some kind of infection. The pandemic and the mass amount of testing taught us that most of the people infected with a respiratory pathogen never develop classic symptoms like a cough, a fever, or shortness of breath. In fact, if you tested yourself every day for a year straight with a full respiratory pathogen panel, you would be astonished at what you'd learn about infection versus symptomatology. You would also discover that when you develop debilitating symptoms, in a lot of cases, you will have a secondary or tertiary infection as well.

In my world, we don't say things like "it's just a cold", we isolate what it is and treat it appropriately. We also record the data so we can pass that along to future generations who want to learn how to handle respiratory pathogens and common illnesses appropriately. I'm not sure if I can emphasize enough how important this one aspect is... We essentially did a case study for the entirety of the world with three years' worth of horizontal data, and the information is so suppressed that we are stifling the advancement of medicine. Not only that, but our lack of understanding of this in the first place is what led to widespread panic and rampant overreaction. The whole world should be screaming for this data to make sure we NEVER go through that again. Suppressing this information almost guarantees that the world will handle this entirely wrongly when something like this happens again.

Testing and Treatment

Stop testing already! We did enough testing during our three-year period. However, when you ARE sick or not feeling well, make sure you get an appropriate test. If you are still seeing a practitioner who does a rapid flu, rapid strep, and rapid Covid test when you go for your visit, FIRE THEM! There are 31 things on a respiratory pathogen panel, and if your practitioner insists on guessing with your health, you should probably guess that they are either churning you in and out because of the volume they need to see to make any money, or they simply haven't a clue about what they are doing. It's highly inappropriate to give you antibiotic resistance because they want to write you an antibiotic immediately to try and appease you and get you out of their office. Respiratory pathogens only take a day to come back, and if a practitioner wants to start you on something that's okay to treat the symptoms, it's a disservice to you if they don't properly identify what illness you have. They can always call you the next day to tell you to stop taking that antibiotic or switch the medication based on your full report. Taking an antibiotic for a virus is useless, and it's a HUGE reason we see a lot of antibiotics not being effective now.

When you understand the science of testing, you come to realize that rapid covid tests are worthless. Throw them out... But if you insist on using them, why are you consistently using them over and over? A rapid test needs a ton of viral load to activate it. It will not give you any inclination as to when Covid is out of your system or even when it is STILL in your system—you're not contagious after 14 days anyway. You could test positive for Covid for up to 90 days on a PCR test, it's just viral shedding. When you insist on consistently using rapid tests, all you ARE doing is wasting your time, money, and everyone else's sanity.

Masks

We don't wear surgical masks for a virus. I saw three people today in the grocery store trying to either "stay safe" or virtue signal. None of the masks they were wearing were N-95 masks, and even if they were, I can almost guarantee that they wouldn't be properly fitted. You are most likely walking around with a Staph infection, and you are more likely to develop Hemophilus Influenza or a host of other bacterial infections. When you test thousands of "mask wearing" subjects over the course of three years, that's what you notice. Just trying to help! I wrote in my first book that masking is the second-stupidest thing I've ever seen in my entire career, I just wanted to reiterate that point.

COVID-19 "Vaccines"

I constantly have to repeat the same line in every media interview I do to let the viewer know what my mindset was at the time when these shots rolled out. That line is, "We never didn't recommend a shot because we thought there would be problems with them. We didn't recommend those shots because, based on the data, you don't need them, and they don't work!" I say that because we weren't going into the rollout with some hypothesis that we wanted to prove or disprove. We were being asked by our patients what our opinion was at that time. I saw enough "fully vaccinated" people coming back Covid positive and saw many of them sick. Also, we didn't lose one single patient to Covid out of our thousands of patients, and only four in total needed any advanced medical care. The obvious recommendation, based on that data, was to NOT get a Covid shot.

Now that these shots have been in circulation for quite some time, we are starting to see the ramifications of rolling out new technology on every man, woman, and child on the planet. Now that we have more data available, these shots have caused massive issues. I'll also reiterate that what you see in VAERS is only scratching the surface. I once hypothesized that only about one percent of cases made it into VAERS. That's a conservative estimate. If you want to give the system the benefit of the doubt, let's hypothesize that as much as five percent of cases could make it into VAERS. With that, take the numbers on the charts being reported and multiply by a factor of 20. The numbers are staggering, and the alarm bells should be ringing. The media should be reporting, and governments worldwide should be screaming for accountability.

The naysayers will always tell you about their own myopic view of themselves or someone they "know". Let's set the record straight once and for all. If you don't know your own CT value or if you have a co-infection, your view wouldn't even be considered in my data set. You may think that the shot made your illness "less virulent" but the truth is, the majority of patients who came before you, when the Covid vaccines didn't exist yet, were most likely less sick than you! In our total data set, only about 10-15 percent of patients even developed a classic symptom. In other words, if we weren't mass testing at nursing homes, police departments, etc., none of those people would have ever been tested for an illness in normal circumstances. We have data from before the shots rolled out, and we have just as much data from the period after the shots rolled out.

The instance of illness or developing a classic symptom is EXACTLY THE SAME!

Your shots didn't make you less sick... To not get sick from Covid was the norm, and your myopic view isn't helping anyone. Those who got the sickest almost always had a co-infection or a very low CT value (high viral load). To those naysayers, your type of "data", the kind where you can't quantify it, only skews the actual clean data to help put COVID-19 into perspective, and I think we have done a good job at that.

The bottom line is, please, stay away from those shots. I have no faith in mRNA technology for mass use. mRNA technology has tremendous implications for the future and in specialties, but remember, these shots were never designed for the whole of the virus. These were designed to only target the spike protein. When Dr. Janci Lindsay reiterated that point during our interview, it gave me pause. Dr. Lindsay stated that this intent could be something nefarious. I can only concur with her statement, considering all the early attempts at rolling these shots out employed the exact same blueprint. Since the early rollouts, only Novavax has developed a traditional shot, much like a flu shot, and that proven technology has yielded much fewer instances of vaccine injury.

On a personal note, I lost four people who very close to me in the last eighteen months. With all the instances of younger deaths and medical anomalies, it makes sense to question the deaths of those around me. I am convinced my father's death had something to do with those shots because his autopsy report was indicative of and very similar to what we see correlated back to vaccine injury. Marilyn's death is also suspect because of her rapid onset of cancer after being screened and cancer-free six months prior to her death. My friend Phil, well, we will never know, but his health was never perfect. In my mother's case, an autopsy was never done, and the medical personnel at the hospital she wound up at did not do the greatest of jobs. I'll never really know if the shots had any long-term effect on her health. What really gets under my skin about my mother is that she bought this narrative and doubled down. She was one of those washing groceries and disinfecting her mail. She wore a mask and stayed at home because of the fear that the government and media used to perpetuate a false narrative. I tried telling her what my team and I were seeing, but you know moms… They never take stock in what their kids say. We weren't close for the latter part of our lives, but we could have been—and that's the kicker.

The years of the pandemic were lost years. They were years we could have spent more time together; they were years when fear didn't have to rule the roost. They were years we could both have lived freely if it weren't for the lies and misdirection. They were years we could have enjoyed rather than be distant. The last real conversation I had with my mother was on her birthday, March 30, 2024. She succumbed to what looked like a brain bleed on June 20, 2024, and later died on June 22, 2024. The last few years, we argued about politics, and she was more than vehement about me getting my "shot" because she wanted me to "stay safe". Of course, I never did because I knew more than her about this subject. However, for her, the media and government narrative was overwhelming and overshadowed anything her son would say, even though I did this for a living… She never read my book to my knowledge, and I found her copy that I had given her when we went through her house. Both my parents listened to the narrative. They both ran out to get their shots and boosters. They both distanced themselves from the rest of us to try and "stay safe" and keep everyone else safe according to the theme of the day. And now they are gone.

Since both of my parents' deaths, I've been contacted by some of my mother's childhood friends. I've made some new friends and acquired photos of my parents that I'd never seen before, and for that, I'm grateful. I've learned more about them in the time they've been gone than I could ever learn during the pandemic years. The time and memories the narrative took away from all of us is atrocious. The sheer fact that we knew all this within the first few weeks of testing and then again within the first few months of the vaccine rollout should make those of you who had your suspicions about this very angry. Anger won't do anything for my parents now. It won't do anything for Phil and Marilyn now either, but it sure can fix things for generations to come if we just have a conversation about what we knew and what we know now. That is how science evolves. Although my mother told me more than once that she was "following the science", little did she know, she was being lied to the entire time.

When we were planning our wedding, my wife Kelly and I decided to take our vows early and on Christmas Eve. My mother came and signed our marriage certificate as a witness. Our ceremony for all our family and friends was months later. When we sent out our invitations, the RSVPs started coming in slowly, but when my mother passed, we still hadn't received hers. When we went through her house, there wasn't a trace of our invitation. I mentioned to Kelly how ironic it would be if it came in the mail posthumously. When all the dust settled and a few days had passed, we got one lone invitation back in the mail. Mom, we are glad to know that you wanted to join us on our special day. We love you and miss you very much...

Acknowledgements

I WOULD LIKE TO ACKNOWLEDGE ALL OUR patients, the patients of my colleagues and the brave men and women who stuck their necks out to tell their stories. Without you, there would be no story to tell! To my wife Kelly, thank you for always having my back. I love you and appreciate all you are! Vincent, you are a very good boy and great company when I write in my chair. You are two for two, get ready for a new project! To my staff, Catilin and all our part-timers, interns, and students current and past, you are valued more than you may know.

On a personal note, thank you to Jaiden Sattler. Keep striving to be the best you can be! To Pat Conway and Jeannie Conway, I love and appreciate you. Thank you, Paul Rotella, Mike Caldarise, and Terry Condio. Thank you, Nick Naumoff and everyone at Rumble. Thank you to the best publicist in the world, Stacy Sutphen at Part Time Hero Productions, you rock! To all our fans of "The Mike Schwartz Show" and "2 Mikes Live", and especially our chat, you all are the best and I appreciate you tuning in every day, despite me butchering your screen names. To Carnella and Joe, thank you for your wisdom and guidance, we miss you. Thank you to my Bats brothers, the NY Yankees, Laura Coreas, Tony Coreas, Larissa Coreas, Fredys Coreas, Victoria Coreas, and Amada Coreas. Thank you, Deb Conrad,

Janci Lindsay, Richard Hirschman, Phil and Marilyn Perricone, Peter Scelfo, Amber May Hilliker, Jeff Ahern, Isaac Hayes, the Bearded Viking Mead Boys, and all the other warriors fighting to tell the TRUTH!

About the Author

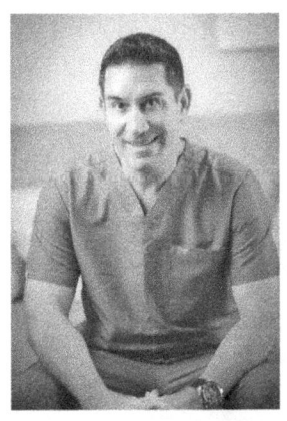

Dr. Michael J Schwartz has been an entrepreneur since 1993. He holds a Doctorate in Business Administration as well as many other degrees, licenses, and certifications. His dissertation is published in the Library of Congress and is centered on how the CARES Act affected testing and treatment of patients during the COVID-19 pandemic. Over the course of his career, he has owned and operated many types of very diverse companies, including multiple medical clinics and a consulting firm that works with physicians and practitioners educating on genetics and respiratory pathogens for immunology. In addition to his duties at Medisure Inc., he also acts as the laboratory director. He is an accomplished private pilot and an avid New York Yankees fan. Schwartz is also a former police officer. He developed and taught a course called "The Secrets of Body Language and Communication" to private and governmental entities. He has been performing stand-up comedy since his early 20s and performs regularly. Michael has appeared on multiple television and radio shows and hosts his own show, "The Mike Schwartz Show", and is the co-host of "2 Mikes Live" on Rumble. He is a contributor to Newsweek and is author of the book *Fauci's Fiction*. Schwartz founded the charity Hometown Heroes in 2008, which is credited with distributing millions in funds to those less fortunate. Hometown Heroes has been recognized by multiple entities and was even awarded the prestigious Robin Hood Service Award. He has sat on numerous boards and has won many distinguished awards for his business career and philanthropic work. He is a recipient of a Paul Harris Fellow from Rotary International. He was recognized by the United Way and received their "Top 40 under 40" award. As a police officer, he was decorated with both a "Class A" and "Class C" meritorious service award. He resides in Wall, New Jersey, and Tampa, Florida.

www.ingramcontent.com/pod-product-compliance
Lightning Source LLC
Chambersburg PA
CBHW020539030426
42337CB00013B/913